Easy Healthy Eating Hacks

By

Rachel Henderson

Acknowledgements

With many thanks to Aly who inspired me to write this book with some fantastic ideas. Also thanks to my husband for looking through the book and contributing a number of ideas.

Contents

Introduction

There is a lot of talk in the media these days about trying to deal with the obesity problem in the UK. This is not just a UK problem of course but something which is spreading across many parts of the world (Stevens et al. 2012). There are many suggestions about what might be causing the problems such as

- Genetics

- Lack of exercise

- Stress

- Lack of sleep

- Poor diet

- Gut bacteria

With so many different theories out there and no one offering a magical pill that will solve it all, it can be very confusing knowing what the best approach is. Some may say that looking at all aspects is important, but from an individual's point of view this can be difficult as we are all busy and it takes time to make new habits in our lives. Looking at what we are eating is probably one of the best places to start though as this is something we can control and it can have a positive effect on our health as well as our size, however, there should be some efforts made towards the others as well.

We tend to hear a lot of things about what to eat and what is healthy or not healthy and although some of the messages are the same, there is also a lot of confusion. This is partly because research studies can show conflicting results, partly because studies might be biased and partly because we are all individuals so have different needs.

There is even some evidence now that our genes can determine what types of foods we can tolerate (Ferguson 2009), meaning that there is not a one size fits all diet. Although it is important to have a basic understanding about food and what is healthy and what is not and there is more detail about this at the end of the book, it can be easier not to get too worried about it all at this stage and later in the book there will be information which should help to clarify some myths. There are a few basic principles which all diets agree on and these can be great way to start. These tend to be:

-        Do not eat junk food

-        Cut down on sugar

-        Reduce processed foods

Although these are quite simple and there are only three, they can actually be difficult to follow without worrying about anything more specific. Therefore this book aims to help with making it easier to follow these rules as well as offering other help too. There are tips and healthy food hacks which aim to help you to have a healthier diet but keeping it really simple. Resisting sugar, junk food and processed foods can be very hard as they are everywhere, taste good, and can sometimes be quite cheap as well. They can feel like a deserved treat and they are also convenient, so give us less work. Sadly, it is these foods that are probably causing health problems for many of us but there are ways that we can reduce these more harmful foods and replace them with healthier foods without having to spend significantly more money or do lots more work.

Healthy Food Hacks and Tips

This section of the book aims to give you a selection of random tips and hacks in order to make your diet healthier but in an easy way. You may already do some of them or have tried some before, but hopefully you will find some new ideas as well that you can consider and hopefully take on.

You do not have to cook!

Many of us will feel tired at the end of the day and feel that we do not have the energy to cook a meal. That is what causes so many of us to get a take-away or put a ready meal in the microwave. This is certainly a lot easier than cooking the same meal ourselves. However, there are ways that we can still have a meal without putting in lots of effort and not turning to unhealthy options.

Find healthy takeaways and ready meals

It could be possible to still have a take away or a ready meal, but to find a healthier option. Look for meals which have less sugar and salt, more portions of vegetables and also think about portion sizes. Take away foods tend to have very large portions and so think about ordering less, keeping half for the next day or sharing with someone. By eating less you will save money and be healthier too. Also, think about what you are ordering. Consider having vegetable and salad side dishes rather than having pudding or lots of rice, potatoes or bread, for example. There are now many takeaways that will offer healthier options and so consider switching to those places, if you have any close to where you live.

When you are buying a ready meal, get into the habit of looking at the nutritional information. There are traffic light warnings on packs these days, showing red for amounts of fat, sugar and salt that are considered to be too high and these can be a quick guide, if you do not have much time. You can also turn over the packs and read the ingredients and look at the nutritional information. The important things to look for are; how much sugar is in the meal, what types of fat are in it, how much salt is in it and how many calories there are. Although I would not recommend rigidly counting calories, if there is a meal which has significantly more calories than another, it could be worth considering the lower calorie option. However, note what has contributed to those calories and what has replaced them in the lower calorie dish. Ideally you want to avoid artificial fats such as margarines and hydrogenated fats and sugary carbohydrates such as white rice, white pasta, sugar and white flour and replace them with vegetables. So for example, when choosing a curry from a supermarket, look for a main course which is lower in sugar and fats and then consider combining it with a vegetable side dish, rather than choosing naan and rice. If you are looking for pizza, perhaps buy half the amount that you would usually have and buy a salad to go with it or buy a plain pizza and top it with extra vegetables yourself, such as peppers, onions and mushrooms.

Have something on toast

If cooking feels like too much hard work then why not just have something on toast? A slice or two of wholemeal toast can be pretty filling, especially if topped with the right things. For a balanced meal top with baked beans and you get two vegetable portions. You can top with cheese if you want to add extra protein and use naturally low in sugar baked beans to keep it even healthier. There is a recipe for baked beans later in the book, which have no added sugar if you want to try something healthier.

Alternatively you can put avocado, pilchards, cheese, mushrooms, or egg on toast to provide some healthy protein. However, you will not get any portions of vegetables this way (unless you choose the mushrooms) but you can always munch on a carrot, a tomato, some cucumber or even lettuce leaves while you are warming up the toast and get some that way. It can feel far less daunting to make a meal like this and there is no reason why it should be any less healthy than a 'proper' cooked meal.

Eat a salad

A salad can be a really great way to get a good range of vegetables without having to cook them. It is, therefore, much quicker, as you just have to do a bit of chopping. You can add a wholemeal roll on the side to get some grains. Put in a hardboiled egg, cheese, tuna or some cooked chicken to add in some protein as well. If you find making a salad too much effort then buy one. Many supermarkets now sell ready prepared salads which have a big range of vegetables and these can be a great alternative to preparing it yourself. They might have slightly less in the way of nutrients as the food may lose some, due to being chopped (Jeffers, 2015), but it is still a far healthier meal than a take away normally would be. They may come with dressings though and these you do need to be careful of. They tend to be either high in sugars or fats or possibly both.

If you do not like salads, then you could just have some vegetable sticks dipped in hummus or guacamole or just have a few salad vegetables but not made into a salad. So if you only like tomatoes and peppers, then just munch on those. It is worth trying all sorts of salads though, we can assume all salads are the same but with different ingredients, dressings and methods of preparing them, we can make many different types. Some people like a pasta or rice salad with vegetables in, some like to roast vegetables and then eat those cold as salad and some like to make herb leaf salads. Experiment with vegetables that you like and you could come up with all sorts of exciting combinations.

Have some porridge

Having cereal for a meal is fine as well, as long as you make a healthy choice. Most cereals are full of salt and sugar and are very processed. Even cereals that are marketed as healthy will often have lots of sugar and processed grains in them. Do not be fooled by those which say no added sugar and then have maple syrup, fruit concentrate or agave in as these can be just as bad as sugar if not worse. All is explained later in the book in the section on sugar.

However, porridge oats are a great cereal to choose. They are just rolled and slightly pre-cooked, so have minimal processing and therefore take the body a lot of effort to break down which means they release energy slowly (Rasane et al., 2015) . You do not even need to cook them, you can just add milk and eat. Adding nuts, seeds and fruit can make it more exciting though! If you do like it cooked, then it is easy to do in the microwave and takes a matter of minutes. If you like granola or muesli rather than oats cooked as porridge it is amazing how easy it is to make. There are recipes for these in the breakfast section, if you want to have a go yourself. If you have some fruit with the porridge, either alongside or in it, you will be getting additional nutrients as well.

Have a sandwich

The poor old sandwich has taken a bit of a battering lately. Many people are giving up gluten or carbohydrates and so the sandwich tends to be demonised as something bad. If you do have a gluten intolerance, then you will obviously need to be very careful with bread and probably avoid it. There are gluten free breads but they tend to be made with highly processed white flour and so be careful what you are choosing. You may find it better to make your own bread. Even if you do not have a gluten intolerance, there are good and bad sandwiches; just like all foods. If you go for a whole grain bread with a filling that includes salad then you can make a healthy alternative to a take away. Something as simple as cheese, lettuce and tomato can be so easy to make and enjoyable but so much healthier than a take away meal. Buying sandwiches can be trickier as they tend to be less healthy than ones that you can make yourself and it really takes very little time to put some fillings between some bread. You can even toast the sandwich to make it feel more like a 'proper' meal.

Make Cooking Fun!

If you have decided that you would like to change your lifestyle so that you are doing more of the cooking, then it is important to make sure that you make this time fun. For some people, it is a great way to relax, to do something different to normal and to slow down and just enjoy preparing the food. For others, they see it as dull and if this is the case then it is important to do what you can to make it more fun for you. Hopefully, preparing a meal, which is nutritious and tastes good will help you to see the preparation as a more positive experience, especially as you get more practiced at it. However, you may find that you want something to keep it more interesting or to keep you entertained.

If you have a television in the kitchen then popping that on, either on a television channel or on the radio can give you something to listen to while you are preparing. If you are the sort of person that gets easily distracted then radio might be a better thing to try because you will not stop and look at the screen in the way that you would with a television program. If you do not have a television in your kitchen then you could use a mobile device to play a radio channel or television show or you could listen to some music or a podcast using one or an MP3 player.

Alternatively, you could use it as an opportunity to sing some songs to yourself while you are getting on. Singing is relaxing for some people and can help to reduce stress levels in those individuals (Daykin et al., 2017). It can also be fun if you like this sort of thing. Alternatively you could recite some poetry or just talk to yourself! You could even ask family members to sit in the kitchen and keep you company, you can chat about your day, help them with homework, do a quiz or something like that while you are cooking to keep things more interesting.

Find Some Good Recipes

It can be really useful to find a selection of good recipes that you and all of the family enjoy. It can take time to practice different things until you find something that you do like. It can help if you have some recipe books or online resources so that you can look up recipes that you like. If you know that you can cook something really good, then you will be more likely to want to do it compared with the alternative options of eating out, ordering food in or buying ready-made meals.

To start with it is good to have a think about what sorts of meals you really like. This could be food that you buy made already, as well as things you have made or that family and friends have made for you. Then you can start to look for recipes for those meals and try cooking them. The great thing about cooking for yourself is that you can tweak recipes so that they taste perfect to you. This could be a case of changing the seasoning on foods or adding more or less of certain ingredients until you get it just right. As you are cooking it is important to taste foods and remember that once you add too much of a seasoning you cannot take it away, so add it little by little until it tastes the way that you want. You will soon get used to how much you like.

Once you find a few recipes that you like, if they are by a certain chef, cook or family member, then it could be wise to try more by them. It is likely that if you like one of the meals that they cook, then you are likely to enjoy more of them.

Prepare meals in advance

If you tend to cook meals, but find that on certain days you are just too exhausted at the end of the day, then be organised. You will possibly know if you have a busy day planned where you are unlikely to have the energy to prepare a meal that evening, so be prepared. If you have time in the morning, then prepare something that you can just warm up later or put something in the slow cooker. If you do not have the time to prepare something then get something out of the freezer to defrost ready to reheat later. It is always good to have a few meals in the freezer as a backup for this sort of situation. It is easy to do this, just cook twice as much food on one day and freeze half. This works particularly well for stews as well as some pasta dishes. It does not take too much extra effort to cook twice as much, but it can save so much time in the future by having food in the freezer to warm up. If you have not been prepared because you were unpredictably busy, then turn to one of the non-cooking hacks above so that you can still have a healthy meal without having to cook at all.

If you are really stuck then you could find some easy choices at your local supermarket or shop that you could grab on your way home to cook. It is easy to make an omelette for example and you can add veggies to make it healthier such as shredded spinach, sliced tomatoes, mushrooms, peppers and spring onions. It will take minutes to prepare them and you can have a tasty quick meal with very little effort. In case you need it, full instructions on how to cook an omelette with some more filling ideas can be found in the recipe section.

Buy pre-chopped veg and salads

Chopping vegetables is something which can be a real chore for some people. While some find it fun and therapeutic, others cannot think of anything more boring! If doing it while watching TV, listening to the radio or listening to a podcast does not make it interesting enough or you just do not have the time to fit it in, then there are ways to get around it.

Most supermarkets sell pre chopped vegetables. These will be more expensive but they can make things a lot easier when you are cooking. A bag of prepared stir fry can cook in minutes and give you a big range of different vegetables with no waste and no chopping. You can buy frozen vegetables which either need no preparation at all such as French beans, peas, sweetcorn, broad beans, broccoli, sprouts and edamame beans or you can buy them already chopped ready for cooking such as onions, butternut squash and roasting mixes. You can even buy vegetables ready to steam in your microwave. These convenience foods are very healthy as they normally have no additives and are frozen very quickly after being picked or prepared, meaning that they can be more nutritious than those sold 'fresh' in some cases (Bouzari, Holstege and Barrett, 2015).

As mentioned before, there will be salads in supermarkets that have been prepared as well. Many of these can be quite simple with a mix of vegetables and maybe some tuna, eggs or cheese. Try to avoid the ones with sugary dressings or white pasta, rice or couscous in. You should still find that there are some that are healthy and will save you a lot of work and time, but still allow you to have a healthy choice.

Keep healthy food in such as frozen veg

It is much easier to prepare healthy meals if you have healthy food at home anyway. If you open the fridge or freezer and there is not much food in there, it will be very difficult to prepare a meal and so will be very tempting to call for a take away. Therefore, make sure that you have food in. If you are not sure when you will use it, buy frozen or tinned vegetables which are perfectly healthy choices but do not have to be used up quickly. Even tinned fruit can be a healthy choice as long as you do not use the syrup or juice that it is stored in.

If you are cooking a dish, then it is really easy to put some frozen veg in with it. You can add it directly into what you are cooking or put a bowl in the microwave to eat with it. Remember that you can add all sorts of flavours to the veg if you are not keen on how they taste. Herbs and spices are great for this, even simply salt and pepper or butter and cheese can help. Just be careful with your salt levels, particularly if you have a health issue, such as high blood pressure, that requires a lower salt intake (He, Li and MacGregor, 2013). Also watch how much fat you are adding to your meal. Often it can be tempting to add lots of butter for flavour, for example, when adding less butter and some extra seasoning could be enough to add flavour without so much fat, which could add unnecessary calories that may lead to weight gain.

Snacking can be a problem for many of us as well. If we know that there are some tasty snacks then we are tempted to go and eat them, perhaps mid-morning or afternoon or while watching television, for example. It is wise, therefore, not to have foods like this in the house but have healthy alternatives in case you do get hungry. There is a snack section later in the book which has plenty of ideas of things that you could snack on which are healthy. However, try not to get into the habit of always snacking at a certain time in the day. Think about whether you really need the food or whether you are just thinking about eating because you are bored, tired, in the habit of eating or craving something sweet or salty. It can be difficult to break a snacking habit, which is why replacing snacks with healthier foods can be a step in the right direction, but trying to avoid snacking as much as possible, can be an even better step.

Avoid Having 'Seconds'

If you like to have seconds when you prepare a meal, then there is a way that you can still have these without eating too much. Cook the right amount of food, so a portion size for each person and then only serve out some of it. Then when you go back for seconds, you will be filling your plate up with the rest of your portion and therefore not overeating. You do need to be careful if there is more than one of you eating. Some may take bigger portions than others and have more than their share or take more of the unhealthier foods. Therefore it could be wise if one person dishes up all of the food to make sure that it is shared fairly.

If you are catering for guests then it is always more difficult to know how much you should cook and therefore when you have seconds there could be a large amount of food left. In this situation, make sure that you still take a small portion the first time and try not to be tempted to eat too much the second time. It can be easier to do this when there are guests as we can be worried that we will look greedy if we eat too much and you may also want to make sure that there is enough food for everyone. If there are leftovers, do not eat them up as soon as the guests have gone but put them in the fridge to eat at your next meal time.

Skip the sugar

Sugar is really being demonised at the moment due to the fact that it causes so many health problems (Evans, 2017). It has no nutrients in it (Lewin, 2017) and therefore adds empty calories to any food that we eat, that has it in. Obviously it does do more than that; it adds texture to baked goods and flavour to everything it is in. It can also help to preserve some foods such as jams and pickles. However, it is added to so many foods that it is extremely easy for us to have far too much of it without even realising. Trying to cut it out all at once can be really tricky as it is something that we are so used to eating. However swapping out some of the foods that we eat, that contain a lot of it, can really help us to be healthier. Some of the foods to cut down on could include:

- Breakfast cereals

- Cakes

- Biscuits

- Puddings

- Bakery products

- Sugary drinks including milkshakes, juices and smoothies

- Sweets and chocolate

These are probably mainly pretty obvious anyway, with regards to them containing sugar, although you may not consider that juices and smoothies could be unhealthy. You may feel that because the sugar is from fruit and the fruit has nutrients in it, that it is healthy and that is something that we are lead to believe by the companies that sell them. However, those sugars in the juices and smoothies can be some of the most harmful to our bodies as explained later in the sugars section.

You may feel that it is all very well missing these things out and wonder what you can replace them with. There is a section on snacks later in the book which could help you to replace those sweets and chocolate as well as those biscuits and cakes. After meals you could have cheese and oatcakes instead of a pudding or just try filling up on the savoury food instead. There are more ideas for healthier puddings later in the book too. Sweet cravings can become a problem, and if this is the case, then try having berries or other fruit when you get them. However, it is good to try to get out of the habit of having sweet foods at the same time each day, perhaps as a pudding or with morning coffee as it will be much harder to get rid of those sweet cravings if you are used to always having something sweet.

Many savoury foods also contain sugar and we need to watch out for these. For example, many tomato based products such as ketchups and pasta sauces will have sugar added to balance the acidity of the tomatoes. You can use passata instead and if you add dried herbs such as oregano or basil, you will find that they will help to mask the acidity and add some natural sweetness. Check the ingredients on foods that you are buying and also look at the nutritional information which will tell you how much sugar there is in a food. Obviously some foods, such as tomatoes, naturally contain sugars but if you compare different brands of tomato sauce, you will see the amount varies depending on how much they add in. If you make your own, then you can more easily control how much sugar you are adding in.

Eat at a Table

Although eating at a table will not necessarily change the type of meal that you are having it can have an effect on how much you eat and how quickly you eat. If you stop what you are doing and sit down at a table to eat food then you will be resting and taking a break. This will not only make you more aware of what you are eating which can help you to avoid snacking later, it can also mean that you will digest your food more slowly and in a healthier way. This is because research has shown that if we eat when we are stressed it affects our digestion and can lead to us putting on more weight (Chatterjee, 2018).

Sometimes we can stand by the fridge and graze or just have a number of snacks rather than a meal. This can lead us to almost feel like we have not had a proper meal even if we have had a lot of food or lots of calories. It may mean that we feel hungrier more quickly, just because we think that we should or that we have not properly registered in our brain that we have eaten because we have not stopped to do so.

Get the Family Involved

It can really help if you get all of the family involved with the cooking. It can feel less of a chore if you are not always doing it on your own. It can also be very good for them to learn how to cook as well, they will then be able to cook for themselves if necessary. If you have young children then you may not want them to be near to the knife or hot cooker until you are confident that they will not hurt themselves. However, there are still jobs that they can help with such as tidying the table and laying it ready for the meal, getting things out of the cupboards for you, washing up and peeling vegetables with a peeler. As you get more confident, you will be able to teach them more things and they will become more useful to you.

Some families will have a rota for cooking and each member takes a turn. This can work for some people, but if there are family members that are reluctant or that do not cook food that the others like, then it can be tricky. Make sure that you think it through before you assign jobs like this. It might be better to give those that are not so good at cooking alternative jobs such as washing up and tidying away afterwards.

It can be helpful if the family give you ideas on what sorts of food they would eat if you cooked it. One of the most frustrating things about cooking is when others do not eat it. It can then feel like all of your efforts are not worth it. If they choose some of the meals then they will hopefully eat it and it will be worthwhile. It is also worth realising that it will take time for them to get used to home cooking. Food that you buy in restaurants, have delivered or buy ready-made can be much higher in salt and sugar than if you make it at home. They may also contain artificial flavourings and other additives that you will not put in it. This means that you will need to get used to a different taste in the food and so it may mean that you have to eat that meal a number of times before you get used to the different flavour. It is always wise to not expect it to taste like someone else's version of the meal but make you own unique version.

Top Tips for Avoiding Junk Food

- Do not keep junk food in the house.
- Avoid having money with you when you go out for a walk or to work if you think you will be tempted to buy junk food.
- Have healthy snacks with you such as nuts and always make time to prepare a packed lunch where relevant.
- Avoid junk food aisles in the supermarket completely and try to ignore those offers on the ends of the aisles, which are usually junk foods.
- Read labels carefully so that you are not buying food that looks healthy but actually is not.
- If snacking is a problem, then go and brush your teeth when you feel like snacking - you will get a sweet hit and you may not be prepared to dirty those teeth with food.
- Ask friends and family that normally give you junk food, to no longer do it. Hopefully they will no longer offer you biscuits with your drinks, slices of cake or puddings. It may take several gentle reminders and some may not like the idea at all, so you may have to get used to politely declining which can be difficult but gets easier once you form a habit of doing so.

-   Try to avoid going in shops that sell junk food (this is very difficult but by avoiding as many as possible you will be helping).
-   Try to avoid thinking of junk food as a treat, but as harmful to your body. It is a treat for your body to nourish it and eat healthy foods. We do not get a burst of energy from foods with less sugar which can make them seem less appealing but is something worth getting used to as slower release energy is much better for us.
-   As you get more used to resisting junk food it gets easier. This could be because we form good habits or because we no longer crave it so much. Possibly because we are not used to being fuelled on unhealthy fats and sugars. So if you can push through the first few weeks and resist then hopefully it will be easier to keep it up as your enthusiasm perhaps drops.

Feeding Children

Although many of us adults (including me!) are fussy eaters, children tend to struggle even more with different foods. Trying to get children to try new foods or eating things that they think they do not like can be a huge battle of wills (this might also be true of partners!) It can make mealtimes a misery for everyone and even something that you may dread. I experienced this with my children who would eat extremely slowly or put so much food in their mouths, a small spoonful at a time, without swallowing it so that they ended up having to spit it out. They would not eat foods if they touched other foods, if they had a sauce on or if they did not know what it was. Therefore getting them to eat healthy food was a huge challenge and I am sure they lived on Weetabix, bananas, potato waffles, biscuits and avocados for about a year! However, I did persevere and they are now much better eaters with one son always keen to try new things and the other being more reserved but will still eat almost all of the foods that I cook him. I tried all sorts of things and although these may not work for you, I thought that sharing them may be useful.

-        I always ate food that I wanted them to eat to try to tempt them although I am not sure if it worked!

-        I tried not to get cross with them when they were being fussy.

-        I made sure I was in a good mood before trying them with new food so I didn't get cross. I noticed that once I lost my temper I could not be gently firm enough to encourage them to eat and shouting never worked.

-        I gave them a plate of food they liked with a small mouthful of new food on a separate plate and asked them to try it before they ate the things they liked. Then we discussed whether they liked or disliked it and why (something we still do now).

-       I kept reintroducing the new food until they were happy enough with it that it could go on their main plate. Sometimes I cooked it in a different way to see if they preferred it.

-       I thought getting them to help me cook might encourage them to eat but it only worked when we baked!

-       I talked to them from a young age about which foods were healthy and which were not.

-       I got them to pick new fruits and vegetables to try from the supermarket and this made them excited about having them although some were disasters but many were liked.

-       As babies I distracted them with television as I spooned food into their mouths, once they were older they had no television on, as it distracted them from feeding themselves.

-       I showed them how I ate foods that I did not like because they were healthy and taught them what I did to hide the flavour such as adding salt, butter or cheese.

-       I encouraged them to eat the foods they did not like so much first so they could get rid of them and then enjoy the rest of the meal.

Eating out

Generally we are eating out more often these days and this means that we have a big selection of temptations from the menu. If we eat out very rarely as a treat then we may not be interested in being healthy, we may just want to enjoy our food. If this is just a few times a year then it is unlikely to have a big impact. However, if we eat out regularly, perhaps monthly or weekly, then the food choices that we make will be having an impact on us and so we need to be more aware of what we are choosing.

It is not always easy to know what is going to be healthy and we cannot always tell what quantities there are of the different foods and how it is going to be cooked. Some menus have calories and other nutritional information which can be more helpful, but there are many that do not. Also calories do not tell us everything, we still have to guess how much sugar is in the food and what type of what was used etc. There are some things that you can do though, to make the meals healthier.

-       If you can, carefully choose where you are eating. Avoid places which have unlimited ice cream desserts, unlimited fizzy drinks or have all you can eat buffets, as these could encourage you to eat more than you need to.

-       Find the place online and check the menu. This will give you a chance to look through the different options. They may have nutritional information online as well, so this could make it easier for you to compare the items. When you are in a restaurant you may feel rushed in deciding what to eat and this could mean that you make an unhealthy choice, so if you look in advance, you will know what the healthier choices are and you will be able to choose more carefully.

-       Go for a starter rather than a pudding as these are usually healthier or just have one course.

-       Consider having a children's meal as these are smaller but beware if they come with a pudding and drink as these may contain lots of sugar which could outweigh the good you are doing by having a smaller portion.

-       Try to find options which have vegetables or salad with them or ask if they can replace the chips/bread/rice with salad or vegetables.

-       Share a meal rather than having a full portion to yourself if you think there will be lots of food or that it will be too indulgent.

-       Do not worry too much about leaving food. It can feel very wasteful to leave food and there is often guilt associated with doing so for a number of reasons, but you should not be eating more than you need or things that you feel are unhealthy. Ask whether it is possible to take home leftovers and then there will be less waste or see if anyone with you wants to eat it.

-       Ask if there are wholegrain versions. This is unlikely with rice or pasta but might be available for bread. If there are not, it may be better to avoid items like this and go with a dish that has quinoa or where the grains can be removed. Think burger without the bun, curry without the rice or soup without the roll, although a pasta dish without the pasta might be pushing things too far!

-       Puddings can be difficult as there will rarely be a healthy option. This means that it can be wise to try to avoid having one altogether, so try to avoid even looking at the puddings menu. If others with you have one, then you could have a coffee instead. This can be really hard though so as an alternative you could share a pudding with someone or see if there is a fruit based pudding or a cheese board.

These will not be entirely healthy as the fruit may be with meringue or have a crumble topping which will have a lot of sugar or served with sugary ice-cream. The cheese could be served with crackers that have white flour. However, these could be better options than others that are available. If someone you are with tries to twist your arm and you are finding it hard not to offend them by refusing just insist that you are full up.

- It is also important to make sure that you are not tempted to have more than you intended. When you go out for a coffee, for example, you will be met with a temptation of cakes and biscuits as well as extra toppings, syrups and cream, for your coffee. Try to just have a coffee and keep it as basic as you can to keep it healthier. An espresso has no milk so is lowest in fat, an Americano is a watered down espresso which can have a dash of milk so that is low in fat too. A cappuccino has milky froth so has more fat but the highest would be a latte which has a lot of milk. You can usually buy coffee in different sizes which would have an effect as well, obviously the smaller the coffee the lower in calories, if you are having milk in it. You can also choose a skinny option which has a lower fat milk, however, although lower in fat and calories this milk is higher in sugar, so it is still not completely innocent. Flavoured coffees have syrups which are high in sugar or sweeteners and these can often be added to frozen drinks and hot chocolate so make sure that you check what you are getting when you order.

Healthy Eating

Diets

So the first thing that many of us will do if we feel that we need to lose weight is to look at a diet. It might be that we decide to follow a specific diet, join a slimming club or vaguely cut down in one area such as low carb or low fat. However, we have all heard that diets do not work and probably know people that have put the weight back on after losing it, using a diet. Research has shown that only three types of diet might work and these are the Mediterranean diet, a low carbohydrate diet and a vegetarian and vegan diet (Kirk, Shulam and Norman, 2014). But we still look to all diets as the answer to losing weight. The reason that we do this is probably because they can work in the short term. Cutting out a particular food group or reducing calorie intake, which is the basis of most diets, will help us to lose some weight in the short term. We will also start off with enthusiasm and so find it easier to eat less, resist the temptations of certain foods and prepare healthy meals. However, after a while we find it more difficult and the enthusiasm wears off, so we no longer want to put in the time to prepare the healthier meals, we give in to temptation and start eating more, so that we are back to eating what we were before. There is also evidence to show that the best diet is one that we think will suit us the best rather than a specific one (Matarese & Pories 2014).

In order to get around this, people talk about making lifestyle changes instead. This can sound a whole lot more daunting though. The idea of giving up your favourite chocolate bars for a few months or years and once you have lost weight going back to having them again seems far more appealing than giving them up for life. Sadly this is why many people will regain a lot of the weight that they lose. They go back to their old lifestyle and this is why they put the weight on in the first place. This is why you do need to make changes which you intend to stick to. This means that you need to make sure that the changes you do make are changes that you know you can stick to. This could mean reducing rather than cutting out, finding healthier alternatives that you enjoy more and trying to change your mind set so you do not think that certain foods are treats and that going without deprives you.

Your Relationship with Food

It is so important to think hard about your relationship with food and how it influences how and what you eat. Many of us have been brought up with unhealthy food being given to us as treats such as sweets, when we are good, cake for our birthday and eating out for Valentine's Day. This means that it is not surprising that we find it difficult to give up these sorts of food, as it feels like we are depriving ourselves of pleasure or reward.

It is good to try to change this viewpoint. Consider what you and your body deserve with regards to healthy food and good nutrition. You do not deserve to have unhealthy foods that will make you overweight, unhealthy and possibly even kill you. We all deserve to have a long and healthy life and in order to achieve this, we need to start to treat ourselves to healthy foods and this can be a really tricky change to make. It can be good to start by identifying foods that we like which are healthy. It might be that you enjoy nuts or avocados, eggs or smoked salmon, olive oil or strawberries. There are so many healthy foods to choose from, if we can at least find one or two that we really enjoy then we already have a treat which we can have without feeling guilty and will do our bodies good.

It is not easy to change to this way of thinking and I still crave bars of chocolate even though I have not eaten any for six months. However, luckily I enjoy carob, so I buy this occasionally instead and the brand I buy has no added sugars or sweeteners and although it is made with palm oil, which I have not found enough evidence to convince me is completely healthy, it allows me to get some pleasure without having to have sugar or sweeteners which cause me to binge eat more and more sweet foods.

We are all different in the things that we crave, enjoy or really want and so we will all need to think about what foods might allow us to feel like we are having an indulgent treat but without having to sacrifice our health.

The more we eat healthy food choices the more we will get used to them and begin to like them more as well. Adding different herbs, spices and seasonings can help us to discover new flavours which can make them tastier as well. It might be hard to imagine that you might like a stir fry and noodles more than a pudding but it is possible!

There is a real freedom in eating food and not feeling guilty. Knowing that you are nourishing your body and mind can make the food more enjoyable. It may feel that you like eating unhealthy food, but if you are honest with yourself do you feel niggles of guilt? Do you feel uncomfortably full? Do you feel a bit nauseous? Do you feel regret? Do you feel like you want to eat even more, even though you know you have had more than enough? Do you go through a craving for sweet foods, then savoury, then sweet, over and over again? All of this goes away when you start eating healthily.

If we can start seeing healthy food as a treat for our bodies then we will have a much better relationship with food. It can help our family and those around us too if we treat them with healthy food instead of unhealthy things.

Willpower

Willpower is also something that many of us struggle with. When we see foods that we like, even if we know that they are unhealthy, we will want them and sometimes even crave them. Cravings can get so bad that they can be all that we think about and so resisting these foods can be almost impossible. We can then end up eating them, not really enjoying them and feeling full of guilt afterwards.

Having strong or weak willpower is something which some people see as the problem of unhealthy eating. I think that a big part of the problem is the marketing of unhealthy foods and how they are everywhere and so it is very difficult to avoid them. Once we see them and start thinking about them we naturally want them. Although there are people trying to change our food environment in this country, so that unhealthy foods are healthier and marketing is restricted, this is unlikely to be a fast process and so we will need to do what we can to avoid them by ourselves.

I am not going to pretend that this will be easy as anyone who has tried to change their eating habits will know that it is not. Partly because we do have habits and may automatically make unhealthy food choices because that is normal for us and partly because unhealthy foods contain fast release energy which gives us a boost that feels good. However, I have always found that taking a step by step approach works better for me. Rather than just trying to make lots of changes at once, doing things one at a time can be much better.

Step by Step Changes

So a step by step approach might work better for some people. There will be some who are happy to completely overhaul their whole lifestyle, make changes all at once and be prepared to work hard at sticking to it. However, most of us will not have the time and energy for doing that and so taking smaller steps will be better. For example, let's say you want to stop taking sugar in your tea. Some people would just cut it out completely and get used to it without. However, for others they may find it easier to slowly cut it down, perhaps reducing it by half a teaspoon a month and then another half for the following month until they are no longer having any. It is good to identify what sort of a person you are. If you want to make lots of dramatic changes all in one go, then read the book and make as many changes as are necessary to help you. Otherwise, read the book and make a couple of changes. Then when you are ready return to the book and pick up a few other tips to make some other changes. Look other books and resources as well and slowly change different parts of your diet and different eating habits until you are happy that you are making the healthiest choices for you. You could even make a list of the changes that you want to make and tick them off as you achieve each one.

Add in vegetables

I realise that there will be people who are reading this that do not like vegetables. They may feel immediately disheartened by the fact that they need to eat more. However, this is a slow, step by step approach and the steps can be taken in a different order and they can done as slowly as you need. Therefore you do not need to start by immediately filling your plates full of vegetables but just by choosing some that you like and eating those more often.

I do find though that the best way to start a new way of eating is not to cut things out but to add things in. This makes it feel like you are not depriving yourself but you start getting more nutrients in your body which makes you feel better and more able to resist temptation. So if you start by adding vegetables then this can be a fantastic start.

Trying lots of different vegetables can be good, as you may not be aware of what you like and dislike. Cooking vegetables in different ways or using different flavourings or dressings with them will change them too. You may remember not liking certain things as a child but our tastes change and there are now different varieties of vegetables which are sweeter and more palatable. For example, I remember Brussels sprouts being very bitter when I was a child, but now my children love them and do not find them bitter at all. So when you do a weekly shop try a new vegetable each time. Also try to add more vegetables on your plate for each meal. Think about adding beans or legumes as these are very nutritious too. You may feel this is a step too far but if you like baked beans in a tin, then you are eating haricot beans and you could use these in a meal that you make. Or you could choose a different bean – there are many others to choose from, with perhaps the red kidney bean being another popular favourite. legumes and lentils also count as vegetables and although you may think they are just for vegans to eat, you may eat a fair amount of chickpeas, if you eat hummus and lentils can be used to thicken soups and stews and so you may have had these as well without even realising it. There are lots of options available and although you can get them all dried and then rehydrate them and cook them, if you want something quick, then just buy them in a tin or pouch and they will cooked and ready to warm up really quickly.

Try not to be overwhelmed by the choice but look at everything that is available and think about what you might like to try. Maybe you just feel like eating carrots to start with because you know you like them. You might then be happy to buy some hummus to dip them in and maybe add in some cucumber as well. Then perhaps you will add some peas to your main meal, some mushrooms with your breakfast and snack on some sweet cherry tomatoes. You do not have to add in lots of exotic vegetables but you may find that these are the ones that you like. Find out how to cook them before you buy them so that you do not waste them and if cooking is not your thing then buy vegetables that you can eat raw.

Hopefully you can start to eat more vegetables each day even if you just increase it by one new vegetable type a week. It is good to start thinking about how you might be able to add vegetables to your meals or snacks. You can start slowly, so just adding in one vegetable a day and then increasing it to two, then perhaps one per meal or something like that. Think of a way that will work for you and once you get into the habit of doing it, it will be easier. Make a chart if that works for you and tally up how many vegetables you have had each day and see if you reach the target that you set yourself. Also note how many new vegetables you have tried and whether you want to try them again or not.

It is really important to not think about 5-a-day as a maximum target to reach in a day but as minimum target. Try to surpass it each day rather than reach it. Also do not get too worried about portion sizes. A portion of veg is large but rather than having 3 tablespoons of peas, which is a portion of peas, why not have one each of peas, sweetcorn and broad beans and you get a much better variety of nutrients, they are just as easy to cook as each other and you can buy them all frozen. Put them altogether to defrost in the microwave, to steam or mix into your sauce or dish you are making and warm through. It is so simple.

Add in fruit

We tend to increase our fruit intake rather than our vegetable intake when we are trying to increase the nutrients in our diet which means that many of us are already eating enough. This is why I have suggested starting with increasing vegetables rather than fruit. It can also be tempting to buy smoothies, juices or dried fruit bars and think that we are being really healthy. However, these are in forms where the sugar is very easily broken down by the body whereas in whole fruits, some of the sugars are trapped in the fibre and therefore it is harder for the body to break down and some do not even get broken down until the gut bacteria do it for us. They are treated in a very different way to the easily accessible sugars in juices which are often turned to fat by liver (Dolson, 2018).

However, having said that, it is still good to have a variety of fruit but just not to overindulge in it. Try different types and go for the ones that are less sweet. So think about berries, green apples, less ripe fruits and have things like ripe bananas, melons and grapes less often. If you really cannot tolerate vegetables, then having fruit is a good alternative but do try some of the sweeter vegetables like carrots and peas and then see if you can get used to more over time rather than always turning to fruit to get your 5-a-day.

Do be careful when you eat fruit though because of the acid damage that fruits can cause to our teeth. Have something alkaline with fruit such as yogurt, cream, nuts or cheese, have it with a meal or swill your mouth with some water when you have finished to clean off the acid. You could always drink some milk afterwards to have a similar effect.

Get a good quality and quantity of sleep

We all know that we function better if we get a good sleep. However, what many of us do not realise is the way that it affects our body. If we do not get enough sleep it has two main effects on us with regards to food. Firstly we crave high energy foods so that we can stay awake and function which is the very food that is unhealthy for us, such as foods high in sugar and unhealthy fats (Speath, Dinges & Goel, 2013). Then when we do eat and drink the body will take more calories from that food probably due to a change in metabolic rate caused by sleep deprivation (Spaeth, Dinges and Goel, 2015) . This sounds rather odd, but the body takes what it needs form the food and if you are tired then it will take more energy from it. This is very useful to help you to function but it means that you will put on weight.

Getting a good night's sleep can be difficult. Many of us go to bed stressed or still doing things and then it is difficult to switch off. Some of us tend to suffer from insomnia anyway and may have no idea why. If we have young children that wake us in the night then it can be tricky to get a good quality of sleep. However, there are things that we can try out to help us to get a better sleep.

-        Do not eat within a few hours of going to bed

-        Try to avoid screens, particularly mobile devices within a few hours of going to bed or at least 30 minutes even for reading because the blue light can disrupt sleep patterns. (You could try a blue light screen filter if you feel you cannot be without your screen)

-        Make sure the bedroom is dark and a comfortable temperature (if you need a light on, then try red light as this is more restful).

-        Do something to help you relax and wind down before bed such as reading and avoid exercising too close to bedtime.

-        Try to go to bed and get up at the same time each day

-        Prioritise sleep as it is a huge help to health

It is not always easy to make changes like this, so introduce them slowly. Consider honestly which might be having an impact on your sleep and have a go and trying to change it. It is not easy, stopping screen use before bed, going without a nightlight or shortening your day by going to bed early but it could mean that you have a lot more energy and are able to achieve more when you are awake as well as feeling better and being able to eat more healthily.

Reduce stress

Stress can also be a big factor that affects our health and what we eat. Many of us eat differently if we are stressed. For some of us we will not eat and then once we feel better we overeat because we are very hungry. Others will eat while they are stressed to try to combat the stress. Eating when stressed is not good as the body is not in a good state for digesting food and it can mean that we put on more weight if we eat when stressed (Greenberg, 2013).

Eating when stressed can be a habit. Some of us find comfort from food from the flavour, the activity of eating, the childhood memories and the feeling of fullness. This can mean that we think that eating food when stressed will make us feel better. This can happen unconsciously, we reach for food when stressed without there being a lot of thought.

Suggesting someone reduce stress is all very well, but knowing how to do it is a different matter. There are whole books on this subject and it can be a complicated thing to do. However, it is worth starting with identifying what stresses us and then trying to either avoid that stress or find a better way to cope with it. Some people find meditation or yoga works; others find exercise or watching a funny TV program works. It is a matter of trying to think about what helps you to relax and incorporating that into your life. If you feel that it is a big problem for you then buy some books about it or talk to your GP as they may be able to arrange some counselling or have other suggestions that could help you.

Start moving more

If you hate the idea of exercise then please do not skip this section. You will hopefully find some ideas that will inspire you and may learn that you are already exercising without realising it!

Some people really enjoy exercise or do a lot as a natural part of the day, perhaps through their job, while exercising their dogs or in other ways. However, there are other people that just do not like the idea of exercise and feel that it just isn't for them. However, exercise can play a really important role in keeping us healthy, as it has many positive influences on the body. It can reduce stress, keep our weight down, reduce type 2 diabetes risk, prevent osteoporosis, help our mental health and improve heart health, to name just a few. It is therefore something which will help all of us and it does not need to be as difficult as you might think.

Although going to the gym, playing team sports, having a personal trainer or going running suit some people, they are not suitable for everyone. It might be that people do not have the time or the confidence to do things like this or their fitness level is not high enough or that they just will not enjoy it. The great thing is that this is not the only way to exercise and there are lots of different things that you can do.

You may not consider walking to be exercise but it certainly is and so if you can just get walking a bit more, you will be helping a lot. If you can do bursts of walking where you raise your heart rate, perhaps by going faster or uphill, then this can be considered to be moderate exercise. Walking isn't the only way to get exercise into your day though. Walking up and down stairs, doing household chores, gardening, chasing after the children and stretches will all help you. It is good to see whether you can find a way to get some exercise into each day, for example, it can brighten up cleaning windows or washing the car if you think about how much healthier you are getting as result!

Switch to whole grains

Many of us enjoy eating cereals, bread, pasta, rice and potatoes as a big part of our meals. Although some people do say we should not have these at all for various reasons such as gluten intolerance, leaky gut, sugars and things like that, there is not normally a reason to give them up completely unless you do have an allergy or intolerance. If you think this is the case then get it checked by a doctor and ask to see a dietitian or nutritionist to get help on making sure that you are still having a balanced diet. The same applies if you have an irritable bowel as switching to whole grains may cause problems and it may be something that you need to do slowly and carefully. However, most people are perfectly able to tolerate whole grain foods.

Of course, you may not know what wholegrain foods are. These are generally when the whole of the grain is used rather than part of it. For example, in white bread, the bran part of the grain is removed before the grain is ground up which is why the flour is white compared with wholegrain flour which is brown in colour from the bran. It still contains the white part but has the grain as well. This is the same with all flour products such as wholemeal pasta and whole grain pastry. Rice is similar too, although you are getting a grain when you buy it rather than something that is ground up, it still has part of it removed in the white version compared to the brown. With oats porridge oats tend to be almost the whole oat but oatmeal is ground oats. Although nothing is taken away during this process, it is easier to digest and therefore not so good for us in a variety of ways compared to a whole oat.

Whole grain products do have a different flavour and texture. It is often the case that those people that are used to having a whole grain product much prefer it as it tastes perhaps more nutty and has more body to it. However, we tend to prefer what we are used to and so it could take time for us to adjust to these different products. Therefore it would be wise to swap over gently. Perhaps start with half and half bread and then try a soft wholemeal loaf. When you buy bread, even whole grain bread, from a supermarket it tends to have quite a lot of white flour in it anyway to keep it softer. To get a completely whole grain bread you may have to go to a bakery. Bakery bread can actually be a lot better anyway as it has less additives and sugar than supermarkets most of the time. Try looking in your local bakery to see what they have, how much they charge and ask them what ingredients their breads have.

With products such as pasta and rice, they will take longer to cook in the wholegrain form. This might be a big disadvantage if you have limited time for cooking. However, there are some things you can do to speed up the cooking time. First thing in the morning soak the rice or pasta in a saucepan of water. Leave it in there until it is time to cook and you will find that it takes a lot less time to cook it. Rice will still take 20 minutes or so but you can buy precooked brown rice with nothing added to it in pouches in the supermarket which you can warm in the microwave. These are a lot more expensive, but definitely much more convenient. It is not the perfect way to eat it but it is still better than eating white rice, takes hardly any time and if it prevents you from having a takeaway with white rice then all the better.

If you are still not sure, then you could always try going half and half with these products too. Boil water and then add some brown pasta and then add white in it (using the cooking times on the packet as a guide). You will then have a chance to try the brown but also have the pasta you already enjoy with it. It is also worth noting that there are different types of rice such as brown long grain, brown basmati, black and red which are all very healthy but have different textures and tastes, so it could be worth trying different ones.

Switching to whole grains can be a long process of experimenting. Take it slowly though and try one new thing at a time so you get used to them.

Swap some snacks

We tend to all snack from time to time, some of us much more than others. We may be led to believe that snacking is good as it balances our blood sugar across the day but it also means that our bodies have to be digesting food for long periods of time and having elevated blood sugar all day may not be the best for our bodies, particularly if we are prone to type 2 diabetes. However, cutting out snacks is very hard, it could be a habit that you have had since childhood. Therefore it is easier to start with swapping snacks to healthier options with the mind-set that you may try to give them up in the future. Later in the book there are loads of healthy snack ideas and so I will not repeat them here, however, I will share some tips on being prepared.

When shopping in the supermarket, even if you are just popping in for a sandwich, there is always the temptation to get something extra, a small treat. The crisps, chocolate bars and fizzy drinks are all really easy to find and very tempting. It can be so difficult to resist them. If you can, go in with determination that you will not get extras to those items that you are going in to buy. Avoid meal deals as they often include a sugary snack. If you are shopping with someone else, ask them to stop you buying these sorts of things. If, even this does not work, then consider online shopping instead. This will eliminate those impulse buys as you will not walk past the confectionary aisle. It can be really tough, if you are with your children and they expect to get a 'treat' every time you shop. I experienced this myself when my son walked past a cake counter and when I said he couldn't have any; he had a full blown tantrum. I learnt a lesson from this very quickly. Having scooped him up under my arm, I got my other son to help me with the basket and did not give in to his demand. I realised though that I would be in for behaviour like this every time we visited, which we tended to do daily. Therefore we started something new. The very next time we went in, I got down on my son's level and explained to both of them that although they were welcome to look at the cakes we would not be buying any that day. I explained that some days we might buy a treat but that would not happen every day. Thankfully this worked a treat, but for years and years afterwards, I warned them every time we went in a supermarket whether or not they would be allowed a treat. Sometimes they would ask me 'can we choose something' and I would always say yes, but sometimes I would say it had to be a vegetable or a fruit, not something unhealthy. Ten years on, they still know that they have to ask and that they may not always get what they want, although I never say no, when they want to try a new vegetable or fruit!

A few ways to gently swap snacks is to try a higher percentage cocoa chocolate which will have less sugar than a regular bar. Start looking at the nutritional information and compare the sugar amount in each bar and choose the lowest. Also go for a smaller bar, which will have less sugar, overall, than a large bar as most people would eat the whole bar regardless of the size. With crisps buy small individual packets, one at a time. This is more expensive but if you buy a multipack, you have the rest in the cupboard to tempt you. Buy a slice of cake or a single cookie rather than a whole cake or a bag and then you will hopefully eat less overall. Also look for the healthier options. We can be easily fooled by good marketing, so rather than believe the message on the pack that claims it is healthy for some reason or another, always check for yourself. Just because something has less sugar or no sugar, has dried fruit added or is whole grain does not mean that it is healthy. It may not even be healthier than other options that look worse. Low fat products are a good example of this.

Many low fat products have extra sugar in, to make them taste better and this could be more harmful than the fat was. It all depends on what specific changes have been made, but just be wary of labelling, as food manufacturers will do anything to get us to buy their product, even if that means bending the truth somewhat.

Check your portion sizes

Another way to be healthier without going without your favourite foods is to make sure that you are not eating too much. It is easy to overeat and hardly even notice until half an hour after the meal when you suddenly feel very full or get indigestion. Sadly we do not always get those full signals while we are eating and so we need to intervene and make sure that we are being careful and aware of what we are having.

Some people suggest that having a smaller plate can be a good way to keep portion sizes down. This is fine if you cook lots of food and then help yourself to what you want and put the leftovers in the fridge, although, you may just go back for seconds if you have a smaller plate. However, most people cook the amount of food that they intend to eat and so whether it is piled high on a small plate or spread over a large plate it should not influence the amount they eat. There may be some psychological effect that the smaller plate looks fuller so you feel more satisfied and so you may to try it to see if it stops you going for pudding or snacks afterwards.

It could be wiser to think about the amount of food that you are cooking, preparing or ordering to start with. Keep those sizes down and then the food is not there to eat and so your portion size will automatically go down. Also if you are having more vegetables you do not need to reduce the portion size of these. You may want to reduce other things on your plate so that you have room for all of the veggies though.

If you do tend to snack and feel that you do not want to stop doing that, then it will not hurt if you have a much smaller meal size as you will be topping up anyway. So, consider whether you could significantly cut down what you are eating during mealtimes, as it is unlikely that you will not feel hungry.

If you are cooking extra food so that you can put a portion in the freezer for later, make sure that you freeze it as soon as possible. Put it in the freezer before you start eating, if you think that you will be tempted to tuck into that, once you finish the portion that you have served up for yourself.

Swap your unhealthy drinks

I am aware that this can be really difficult. If you are used to having fruit juices, squash, fizzy drinks, smoothies or things like this, then changing them for alternatives can be tricky. There are some things that may make it easier though.

Switching to tea or coffee can be a way to still get drinks without all the sugar. If you are concerned about the caffeine then there are decaffeinated versions which taste very similar and most are decaffeinated using a water method which has no chemicals but even those that use chemicals have to remove all traces of those chemicals before they are allowed to sell the product. There are naturally caffeine free alternatives, such as herb and fruit teas (watch the sugar in these though) and coffee replacements such as chicory.

Some people only like cold drinks though and so replacing them with milk or water could be an option. Obviously water has no taste and although lots of people do drink a lot of it, some people find it unpalatable. You could try adding a small amount of lemon juice or some other fruit such as strawberries into the water to flavour but this will add sugar and acid which could harm your teeth and give you a sweet tooth! Try it warm, boiled, room temperature, with ice and even fizzy to see if any of these appeal to you. You could try brewing green, fruit or herb teas and then leaving them to cool and serving with ice. To make milk more exciting you could add a shot of coffee and pour over ice to make a coffee milkshake or even put in a blender to make it frothy. Do watch out if you switch to drinking a lot of milk though. Milk has natural sugars in it which are higher in the lower fat versions, so you need to be careful if you are drinking more of it, especially if you are carefully watching your weight or your sugar intake. The fat will also add calories to your diet; perhaps more than the alternatives did before. Plant milks can be seen as a healthier alternative but you need to be careful. Some may be lower in fat, but they often have added sugar so you may want to compare the nutritional information to make the best choice for you. Of course, plant milks vary a lot in flavour too and so you will want to take that into account as well.

It can take a long time to adjust to drinking something different. When my father gave up having sugar in his tea and coffee he said it took him a year to enjoy a drink. When I went through a time of not drinking dairy, I did not drink tea at all, as I did not like the taste without cow's milk in it. It is worth experimenting with different drinks though, as you could find that you really like a particular healthy alternative that you never thought you would.

You may find that you need to make changes slowly. If you are used to drinking coke, for example, then it can take time to get used to not having that caffeine and sugar at regular intervals through the day. Some people find it easier to swap to a sugar free version first and then reduce the amount, some just cut out completely all in one go and others cut down slowly so they get more used to it. You need to find a method which works for you.

Change your breakfast cereal

Many of us will eat breakfast cereal first thing in the morning. It is very convenient and there are so many options that we are bound to find one that we enjoy the taste of. Some of us will also snack on cereal or have a bowl for another meal or instead of a pudding. However many cereals are unhealthy, with sugars, processed grains and salt in them in high quantities. It can be something which is difficult to change though.

Later in the book you will find breakfast ideas and recipes to try but making this step is difficult. Moving away from pouring a bowl of cereal, slopping on some milk and quickly eating it each morning can be difficult. At the weekends we may have more time and so this could be a good chance to try some different breakfasts. You may find that you discover one that is quick enough to make on a weekday morning and much healthier.

If you are sticking with cereal it is worth checking ingredients and nutritional information to see whether you are making a healthier choice. It can be easy to be fooled as something which states it has multi-grains and less sugar might seem great. However multi-grain does not mean whole grain it just means that there a bigger variety of white flour in it, rather than just wheat. Although having a variety of different grains is good, once the grain has the outside removed most of the nutrients are removed with it, the benefit of having more than one grain may not be there at all. Also it may have less sugar than another cereal in their range but it does not mean that it will be healthy. Comparing sugars in the nutritional information can be tricky though. If the cereal has fruit then that will add to the sugar content and some people would claim that the fruit is a healthily sugar and therefore should not be counted. However, it will be dried fruit which has very concentrated fructose that is easily available unlike fruit, in its natural state, when the sugars are less easily available. Therefore it is safer to just count it as the same as any other sugars when comparing percentages.

Even the cereals branded as healthy can be confusing such as the expensive granolas and mueslis which are labelled sugar free but have a variety of fruit concentrates and syrups to sweeten them which can be less healthy than sugar itself. It can be so much better to make your own muesli or granola and there are recipes later in the book to show you how. It may seem hard, but actually it is very quick and simple and you can add ingredients that you enjoy and leave out those that you do not.

Reduce your sugar

It is worth looking at the sugar content of all of the foods that you are eating as well as cereals. Hopefully you can swap out unhealthy sugary snacks and cereals but sugar does seem to crop up in many foods and can be really hard to avoid having. Puddings might be an area where you have a lot of sugar and could be an area to look into changing. You may also find it hard to resist those sugary snacks. Below are a few tips that might help you:

-	Share your pudding with someone else so instead of having a slice of cheesecake each, have half each and then you will still be able to have some, but you will be halving the sugar that you are having. Once you get used to that, see if you can reduce it even more, perhaps by just having a quarter.

-	Change your chocolate to a higher cocoa version as these have less sugar in. Look at the ingredients and it should say what percentage of cocoa solids there are in the bar. Gradually increase that percentage and you will be gradually reducing the sugar that you are having. Also buy small bars and just buy one bar at a time, so you do not eat too much.

-        Practice saying 'no thank you' when a friend or relative offers you a biscuit or cake when you visit them. This can be harder than it seems as you may just automatically take one and find you have eaten it before thinking about the fact that you should be trying to cut down. Some people can be very persuasive, so try to be prepared for this, perhaps by saying you are full or asking for a healthier alternative, then they may not push you so hard towards the unhealthy item. You could even offer to bring your own healthier alternatives when you next visit.

-        Try to get all of the family on board because if they are eating sugary foods you will be tempted by them and it will do them good to have them less often.

-        Have a think about how you can replace the sugary foods that you like with healthier options. This is easier with savoury foods that have hidden sugars such as replacing a pasta sauce with passata or baked beans with a sugar free version as you almost have a like for like swap. Finding a replacement for a cake, biscuit or sweet is not so easy but it is possible. You could try making your own sugar free versions, swap for savoury foods such as having cheese scones instead of sweet ones or a buttered oatcake or some wholemeal toast instead of a biscuit. Do watch out though as some savoury items can have as much sugar in as sweet items.

Check your fats

Fats are no longer seen in the same light as they used to be. You may remember when all fats were considered to be bad and low fat diets launched. Then there was a change of heart with some fats being considered worse than others and this tends to be the current thinking although ideas on which are healthy may have changed. This means that you may need to think about changing the fats in your diet.

Deep fat fried foods might be really tasty but unfortunately are still not good for us regardless of which fats are used. This is partly because of the high calories in the fat which can make us gain weight. This means that we should be really careful with how many of these items we are having. We may not have deep fat fryers or chip pans at home but when eating out it can be really easy to have a lot of deep fried foods such as chips, sweet potato fries, chicken nuggets, deep fried halloumi, tempura vegetables, onion rings and things like this. If it is battered or bread crumbed then it is likely that it has been deep fried so try to avoid these or have less of them if you can.

Having fat with our meals is important though, as it helps us to absorb the fat soluble vitamins such as Omega 3 and vitamin D. A lot of the time though, we will not have to add extra fat as it is already in the food, so if we have fish, meat, dairy, nuts, avocado, or seeds then we will already be getting enough fat in that meal.

Cooking in fat can be problematic. If the fat burns, then it can be carcinogenic (Grootveld, Percival & Grootveld, 2018) and if we have a lot of seed oils then we are getting too much omega 6 (Simopoulos, 2016). Therefore be wary of cooking with too much fat and try to choose healthier fats such as olive oil. Try not to heat food up to too high a temperature either. This is more easily done when grilling, barbecuing or frying rather than the oven. Although the oven temperature seems high, it will not go too high, unlike when frying, when the pan can just get hotter and hotter and start to smoke. I try to fry with some water and oil in the pan and keep the temperature low to stop it smoking.

It can be worth looking at any items that you buy to see what types of fat are in them. Although I tend not to worry about the amount of fat or whether it is saturated or not I do like to see what fat is used. I try to avoid things which are high in seed oils because of the omega 6. Anything which has hydrogenated fats I also avoid as these are artificial and unhealthy. I also avoid things with mono and di-glycerides of fatty acids in them. This is a big mouthful but basically it is a lab manufactured product which hardens fats and makes them have a longer shelf life but it is a type of trans-fat which we should be avoiding, as they have been proved to be very dangerous to heart health (Mozaffarian et al., 2006). Trans-fats are regulated and not allowed to be in products at more than 1% but as ingredients that are less than 1% do not need to be listed then they could be in lots of things. If we are also having these mono- and diglycerides then we could be having a lot more trans-fat than we realise.

Healthy choices

The words 'healthy choices' are rather tricky to interpret and can be bewildering. We are given so much health advice and if we try to research and find out what is healthiest for us, much of it seems to contradict itself and that can be extremely confusing. Although evidence is not changing a great deal, information can be presented in different ways to suit different people so it is possible to use the same data to support completely different viewpoints and even doctors get it wrong. I am confused as well, but from all of the different books, articles and research data I have seen, I have pulled together some information which I share below. I am not afraid to admit that there are places where I am confused as well and suspect that more research may show my current thoughts to be incorrect which has happened in the past. For example, being brought up in an age when low fat diets were seen to be the best I decided that a vegan diet, almost free from saturated fat was really healthy. But now I understand more about nutrition, I am not convinced that it is the healthiest diet, although it does have many components of a healthy one if you are careful in what you eat.

Another confusing thing is when manufacturers label their food to imply that it is healthy. It can be so easy to be fooled by them as they work really hard to sell their products. They might make claims like:

- Low in fat

- Multigrain

- No added sugar

- Low calorie

- High in fibre

However, none of these necessarily make a product healthy. Many low fat products have extra sugars added to make them tastier or they have unhealthy fats in them. If something is multigrain it may have more of a variety of grains but they may not be whole grains and therefore not much healthier. If a product claims there is no added sugar, it may be high in naturally occurring sugars or may have syrups or sweeteners added instead. If something is low in calorie it might have the fat removed and replaced with sugars, it may be a tiny portion or it might be made up of all sorts of artificial ingredients. If something says it is high in fibre it may have inulin added, which is a type of plant fibre but does not mean that it is any better for you with regards to fats and sugars.

Using manufacturers as a guide to whether products are healthy can be extremely confusing. They will make all sorts of claims to tempt you and they do not always mean anything. The best way to find out what is really going on is to look at the ingredients. You could find that there are all sorts of ingredients with long names that you have never heard of and these could be anything. Some people say that it is best to only eat foods that your grandmother could recognise the name of and there is some sense in this as you will not be having artificial foods. However, not all of our grandmothers ate healthily, I know one of mine had puddings each day, indulged in sweets when they could afford to and did not have a big variety of fruit or vegetables. She also spent most of her life on a diet, but I always remember her being overweight and she ended up with type 2 diabetes.

It can be easier to break food down into main groups and discuss them to find out more about them. Then you will get an understanding of what makes up different foods and how you can make them healthier.

Food Types

Fats

As I said before fats used to be the enemy. We were told that all fat was bad for us as fat made us fat. Although this seemed to make sense, everything we eat has the potential to make us fat and there are some positives to eating fat. Fat is essential for us to thrive and there are some vitamins that are only absorbed in fat and so if we eat them in a meal without enough fat our body cannot absorb them. However, this is not an excuse to eat as much fat as you can! There are different types of fats, as most of us are aware and some are better for us than others.

We used to be told a lot about saturated and unsaturated fats. The fats that are solid at room temperature contain mainly saturated fats (such as lard, butter and coconut oil) and these were thought to be worse than the fats that were mainly unsaturated such as vegetable, seed and olive oils. However, now the thinking has changed slightly in that some people are saying there is not such a strong link between fats and illness as was first thought but there are some specific fats which are unhealthy.

Trans-fats are usually artificially made fats, although they do occur naturally in a few products. The process is quite complex but simply put an unsaturated fat is made into a hard fat usually by a laboratory process. This forms what is called a trans-fat and research has conclusively shown that these are very bad for our health. (Mozaffarian, 2006). These are not put in large quantities in food anymore because people are aware of the health problems they cause. However, they can be put in foods and not listed on the ingredients if they are in tiny amounts. They are also in mono-and diglycerides of fatty acids which is an emulsifier used in a lot of processed foods. Therefore there is a chance that they could be present in some processed foods, margarines and spreads, pastries, pies and things like this. I have also seen evidence that it may also appear in deep fried foods where the oils are reused, such as in restaurants and takeaways (Grootveld, Percival & Grootveld, 2018). It is best to avoid eating these as much as you can.

Many people now feel that naturally occurring fats are better for us, so those in nuts, seeds, avocados, fish, dairy and meat compared to those that have been refined and processed such as margarines and spreads and those in processed foods. Research has even shown that dairy fats do not have such a bad influence on cholesterol levels than it was once thought and in fact they may have no effect at all (German et al, 2009). Avoiding processed foods can have a lot of other advantages with regards to our health and these will be explained through the book.

It seems to be agreed that omega 3 fats are really healthy for us particularly for our hearts and brains. If you eat fish then having oily fish a few times a week can give you enough. However, many people do not eat fish and so look for alternatives. Walnuts can be a good alternative and many other nuts and seeds also contain omega 3. However, omega 3 needs to be taken in the correct proportion with omega 6 to be effective and in seed oils such as sunflower, these are not in a good proportion, with too much omega 6 meaning that the omega 3 is not available to the body (Simopoulos, 2016). Some people prefer to take supplements if they do not like fish. There are fish oil supplements but if you do not eat for ethical or allergy reasons, then you can take algae omega 3 supplements which claim to be as effective. Other alternatives, such as those with the omega oils from flax seeds may have too much omega 6 in them, so be careful when you are making your choice.

Sugar

We have probably all heard about the warnings with regards to us eating more sugar than we should. Sugar is very hard to avoid though, unless you are cooking everything from scratch. This is because it is added to lots of foods, both sweet and savoury and it can be almost impossible to avoid it completely. Even trying to keep below the maximum recommended amount can be extremely difficult.

It is worth understanding a bit about sugar and why it is so important that we are careful with how much we eat. Many people think that it is just to do with calories and that as sugar is considered to be empty calories then we should not eat it. Although this is true, like the problems that sugar can cause for our teeth, there are other reasons that we should be wary of it as well.

Firstly there is a risk of type 2 diabetes in those people that eat a lot of sugar. This is because when we eat anything, our body responds by making sure that the amount of sugar in the blood is regulated. This means that if there is too much sugar in the blood, the body sends out a signal, using the hormone insulin, to let the body know that the sugar should be absorbed into parts of the body and stored as fat. However, if the insulin is being produced a lot, because there is a lot of sugar being consumed, then the cells ignore the warning and stop taking up sugar when they are instructed to. This means that the sugar remains in the blood stream where it can do damage. This is a complex process which I have over simplified but hopefully it can help you to understand why having too much sugar in the body can lead to a condition known as insulin resistance which is a precursor to type 2 diabetes. Type 2 diabetes can lead to all sorts of problems with the body such as blindness, losing limbs and there are even now seen to be links with dementia (Biessels et al. 2006). Therefore if we can reduce the sugar in our blood we can help to prevent this situation.

It is important though to understand what is classed as a sugar or at least what is treated as a sugar by the body. There are many different types of sugar and anything that is called a syrup or has –ose on the end of it in the ingredients list is a sugar. However, food manufacturers are getting clever at calling things different names to make it harder to identify that they are sugars. We also have the confusion of sugar substitutes which are classed as being better for us, when some of them are not. Things like maple syrup, coconut blossom nectar and agave are used in many recipes as a 'healthy' alternative. There are advantages in that they will not cause an insulin release and therefore do not contribute to insulin resistance. This sounds great as at the moment research seems to show that they will not damage our bodies in this way. However, the type of sugar in them is called fructose and this is metabolised by the body in a very different way to other sugars, such a table sugar, glucose and lactose (which is found in milk) rather than being burnt off when needed and then stored as external fat when not needed, fructose is sent straight to the liver and metabolised there (Maersk, et al. 2012). The liver turns it straight to fat which sticks around the liver and other internal organs and causes non-alcoholic fatty liver disease. This can increase your risk of heart disease, strokes and diabetes as well as cirrhosis of the liver.

Therefore we need to be extremely careful with the foods that we are consuming that contain fructose. When diabetic foods first came onto the market they would contain fructose instead of sucrose but now more is understood about it and artificial sweeteners tend to be used instead. Foods that are high in fructose include fruit juices, smoothies, dried fruit, fruit bars, jam, snack bars containing maple syrup or agave and honey. Honey sometimes has a lower amount of fructose in, but it depends on the specific honey that you buy as to how much it has. Fruit and vegetables also contain fructose but it is harder for the body to get it out. It can be trapped within the fibre in them and so the body does not release it but it gets digested by the gut bacteria and therefore not by the liver (Pinnock, 2018). Some fructose will be released through chewing but if you avoid the fruit juices and smoothies, dried fruits and things with added fructose, then you will be a lot better off. This can be confusing as we are told that fruit juice/smoothies can be part of our '5-a-day' and they are marketed to us as a good way to get lots of nutrients. However, we can get nutrients from the whole fruit and in fact the skin often has more nutrients in and vegetables tend to be more nutritious than fruit.

Sweeteners are also something which have been controversial over the years. These can often be used to replace sugar, such as in diet drinks. These have some beneficial effects, but they are not as good as they may seem. Although they will lower calorie intake because they are often zero calories compared to sugar, having a calorific value and they will not spike blood sugar because they have no sugar in them to cause that spike, they have been found to have detrimental effects as well. Studies have shown that aspartame can lead to the destruction of gut bacteria (Pretorius 2012) and that sweeteners can also change the gut microbiome leading to glucose intolerance which is often the precursor to type 2 diabetes (Suez et al. 2014).

Carbohydrates

Although sugar is a form of carbohydrate, I have given it its own section above as there is so much to explain about it. Carbohydrates are usually thought to be starchy foods which are often grains such as wheat, rye and barley or vegetables such as potatoes and plantains. However, fruit and vegetables are also carbohydrates as are sugars. However, we will discuss vegetables and fruit in a separate section below so here we will concentrate on the grains.

In the UK we tend to mainly eat grains as flour in foods such as bread, pasta and pastry. We eat some grains in a more whole form such as oats and rice. The way we process grains will affect the impact that they have on the body. Many grains are polished to remove the husk which is the fibre in the grain and the part which also contains most of the nutrients. However, it is possible to buy most grains in a more whole form. Oats are just rolled whole oats and therefore are in a very fibrous form. Brown rice is not polished and therefore contains the more nutritious and fibrous outer casing. Whole grain flours contain the whole of the grain and so if you cook with these you have a more nutritious product than if you use a 'white' option. When it comes to more processed forms such as bread and pastry then it is not always easy to find whole grain versions. Even wholemeal bread contains some white and some wholemeal flour; even though the ingredients say it is wholegrain. Therefore you may want to make your own bread or source it from a bakery which uses all wholegrain flour in the loaf. When you grind a grain into flour it makes it easy to digest which means that it is easier for the body to get at the sugars in it and it has less fibre and therefore it is not so good for us. Many of the nutrients re also contained in the part of the grain that is removed. Therefore going for whole grain options and choosing coarse ground flour or using some of the complete grains within the product is a healthier option.

Many people have chosen to try removing carbohydrates from their diet. Although this can lead to rapid weight loss it can be rather extreme and means that you do not have so much fibre in your diet. It can also be difficult to stick to in the long term as the variety of foods available is lower and so it can get boring. Reducing the amount of sugars will help with weight loss and to keep away diabetes but you need to get a good balance. As you will see later, vegetables particularly have lots essential nutrients in them and whole grains are also a nutritious part of our diet. If you are a vegan, for example whole grains provide essential proteins which you may need in your diet, depending on what others foods you also eat.

Vegetables and fruit

There is no diet which doesn't recommend that we eat lots of vegetables. Even a paleo diet, which is mainly based on fats and proteins, will still recommend having vegetables and in fact hunter gatherers tend to have about 80% of their diet made up of fruit and vegetables. Therefore there is really no reason why we should think that eating vegetables is not doing us good and in fact there is a lot of evidence to show that they actually contain a lot of nutrients which do keep us healthy.

Most of us are aware that fruit and vegetables have healthy vitamins in them and they also have minerals as well. A lot of these are essential which means that the body cannot make them and so we have to consume them in order to keep the body functioning normally. They also have fibre in them which is something that we have been told help things moving along the gut. Although this is true, in the last decade or so research has shown that the fibre also helps to feed our gut bacteria. (Pinnock, 2018) These are in everyone's bodies and they will digest the food that we cannot, such as the fibre from plants. This is good for us because those bacteria then produce hormones and nutrients which we use in our bodies so we need to keep them happy in order to keep us healthy. Vegetables can also contain some protein, particularly beans, peas and lentils and eaten together with grains or nuts can provide enough protein for us without having to eat dairy, eggs, meat or fish, which is important for vegans who do not eat these.

In the UK we are told to eat 5-a-day but other countries have much higher recommendations. This is probably because if the target is really high then people may decide not even to try as they will not reach it. I see it more as a minimum rather than a maximum and try to have at least ten if not more different fruits and vegetables in the day but not necessarily in massive amounts. Then I am getting a good variety and it is more interesting than eating the same things but also gives me good range of different nutrients.

This can be daunting though, especially if you are not a big vegetable and fruit eater. Remember the step by step plan and slowly introduce more into your diet to make it easier. Try lots of different vegetables and fruits so that you get to know which ones you like the best. If you find vegetables boring then make sure you have sauces, gravies and dressings to go on them – they do not have to be boring! At the end of the book is a section all about vegetables and different ways to eat them to give you some ideas on how you can choose the best vegetables for you to eat and how you can prepare them to make them taste good.

Meat and fish

With the growth of veganism and the health messages running alongside that, the warnings about having too much red and processed meats but dietary advice stating we should have oily fish it can be really confusing knowing whether we should eat meat and fish and how much we should eat. Even experts cannot really agree but there are some things that you can consider changing to make sure that you are eating them healthily.

Firstly to deal with the processed meats that have been linked with cancer. If you actually look at the stats they are a risk but a small one. However, processed meats will often come with other foods that are unhealthy. Such as pasties, sausage rolls, pork pies, chorizo pizza and things like this. It has occurred to me that the risks of eating processed foods may be partly to do with the way that we eat them rather than the meat itself. However, keeping them down to a minimum is probably a good idea. So although bacon and sausages are processed and may come without these unhealthy accompaniments, it is probably sensible to not have them frequently. If you are given them when eating at someone's house then do not feel that you have to be rude and decline them but consider whether you really should be buying them to consume at home.

Red meat has also had some negative press whereas white meat tends to fair better because it is less fatty. However, messages about fat have also changed recently too so it is really hard to know what to do for the best. I tend to restrict my family to having meat on special occasions or when we are eating out. Then they still benefit from the iron and protein in the meat but they do not have a high risk of the negative health effects. I suspect that there will changes again in the attitude towards meat in the next few decades and I am interested in seeing what research is being done and what conclusions are being drawn. I may change my mind about it but at the moment when I buy meat to cook at home I choose the best quality that I can and although that is expensive it is purchased so rarely it becomes affordable.

Fish is a different matter with health benefits of oily fish with regards to the omega 3 being talked about a lot and white fish for its iodine. However, there have been problems with fish having mercury and lead in due to the poisoning of the oceans and more recently there has been talk about plastics in fish. This means that recommendations tend to be that we eat smaller fish that are lower down in the food chain. They have less chance of ingesting so much poison and plastic. Also the source of the fish can make a difference so this could be worth researching if you do eat a lot of fish.

We are advised to eat oily fish twice a week for the omega 3 benefits to our hearts and brains (NHS, 2017) and also to have white fish weekly as well. A lot of people do not like the taste of fish or cannot tolerate oily fish or choose not to eat fish due to being vegetarian. If this is the case then it is important to ensure you get your omega 3 elsewhere, perhaps from algae supplements or from walnuts. Iodine can be got from vegetables that are grown near the coast and from dairy but vegans may want to supplement, although if you have any thyroid problems you would need to speak to your doctor first.

Protein

There is a lot of talk about protein as well, how much we need and that we should be having more if we want to build muscle and things like this. It is worth understanding a bit about protein first.

Protein is not something that we can eat, our body makes it using amino acids which we get from food. There are lots of different amino acids that we need and some foods contain all of them and some contain just a few. For example meat, fish and dairy contain all amino acid groups in good quantities. However, if you do not eat these products, then you will need to find them elsewhere. Nuts and grains are high in certain types of amino acids and beans and pulses are high in others which means that if you make sure that you have grains or nuts combined with beans or pulses then you get enough of the amino acid groups to form all of the protein that you need. There are some vegan foods that do contain high quantities of all of the amino acid groups and these are quinoa and soya.

We usually get enough protein in our diets and even if we are trying to build muscle we are probably getting enough from what we eat. If we do take on protein powders or bars we are probably just not using all of it. There are cases of protein deficiency but only among communities that are experiencing famine or among people who have a highly restricted diet, where it is still very rare.

Some people do believe that it is actually unhealthy to have too much protein (Rabin, 2016). This is probably unlikely to happen to anyone following a balanced diet but it is worth considering how much you are having, particularly if you are supplementing with it, to be sure that you are having safe levels.

Dairy

It is easy to get really confused about whether dairy is good for us or not. We can sometimes see headlines which claim it is good for us and others which claim that it is bad. There are lots of low fat dairy options which we might think are better for us, but then others will say that we should be having full fat to avoid the sugar in the lower fat products. Then there is the massive growth of plant milks and many claims that these are very much better for us. Some people also feel better if they avoid dairy. So what should we believe and what should we be doing?

If you think you have an intolerance to dairy, perhaps lactose intolerance or dairy allergy then speak to your GP. They will be able to let you know whether it is something that you might have. If you do think that you feel better when you are not eating dairy, then speak to them about it. They should be able to give you some ideas for alternatives that will ensure that you continue to get a healthy diet. Vegans choose to give up dairy for ethical reasons. If you do this then make sure that you find out about how to replace it in your diet. If you would rather not see a doctor, then you will find that there are vegan websites which have this information for you.

It is often the fat in dairy products that is criticised to be bad for health. However, if you are worried about cholesterol then the fat in dairy does not harm it but it does not help it either (Jephcote, 2018). Therefore this should not be a worry, but do check with your doctor if you have been told to avoid dairy to reduce your cholesterol levels. The problem with all fats is that they are high in calories and so you do need to be careful about how much you have if you are trying to lose weight. They can also contain a lot of sugar and so you need be wary of that. Milk contains lactose, which is a form of sugar and this is higher in skimmed milk than whole milk. There is very little in butter or hard cheeses, but comparatively more in soft cheeses, cream and yogurt. Although you may need to be wary of this sugar, it tends to be processed dairy foods that have even more. I am referring to flavoured yogurts, milkshakes, cheesecake, some coffee drinks, custard and things like this.

Alcohol

Although not a food, it is worth having a think about alcohol. It is something which most people consume and it is becoming more common to drink alcohol in the home, rather than only when out for meal or in a pub or club.

Most people are aware that drinking too much can alter our behaviour and slow our reactions which is why it is illegal to drink more than a certain amount and then drive. These behaviour changes are the reason that some people drink as they feel more relaxed or confident than when they do not. It can also be a social thing, where when groups of people get together they have a drink together and so it feels like you are being rude if you do not have a drink with them.

It is worth understanding a bit more about alcohol though. It is a poison to the body. The liver has to remove the toxins and this causes stress on it. This is why heavy drinkers can get a disease in the liver which actually damages and permanently destroys part of it (NHS, 2018). People who do not drink heavily may think that they are safe from this but there are other diseases also associated with drinking such as many types of cancer (Cancer Research UK, 2018).

We also get resistant to the effects of alcohol on the body. This means that if we want to feel different as a result of drinking alcohol, we may need to drink more and more to get the same feeling. This could mean that we end up drinking quite heavily and we may even realise that we are increasing how much we are drinking until we stop and add up how many bottles or cans we are buying each week compared to how many we used to.

Some people may feel that the stress relief they get from drinking is worth the risks to their health. However, it could be worth trying to replace those alcoholic drinks with a different form of stress relief which could be as effective if not more so and better for your health.

It can be good to add up how much you are spending on alcohol as well, because you could find that you would save a significant amount of money if you cut down or cut it out and so you will get additional benefits as well as those benefits to your health.

Meal Ideas

The meal ideas are not all recipes and they all aim to be as simple as possible. The point is not to necessarily follow each exactly but to take away some ideas and then adapt them to suit your needs. There are ideas for all types of meals including snacks, which is where it will start as it is probably an area where most people need some help.

Snacks

When we snack we want a quick convenience food that will fill us up until our next meal. It can often be something we will also feed to our children, perhaps more often than we feed to ourselves and this means that it is important for them to be even healthier as we will want our children to grow up with healthy habits. Alternatively it can be something we take with us when we are out and about. Often we can be tempted to buy unhealthy snacks when we are out, perhaps chocolate bars from the vending machine at work or ice-creams when we are out with the children. We often turn to choices which are not healthy even when we are in the home but there are many things that we can try which will help to fill us up without being unhealthy. it can be wise to keep healthy snacks in the home and get into the habit of keeping them with you, whether that is in the car, in your bag or in your desk so that you are not tempted to have something unhealthy instead.

Start with a drink

There are people that say that we feel hungry when we are actually thirsty and so we should have a drink rather than food. To me this does not make a lot of sense, as I can tell when I am thirsty and when I am hungry and so why would the body sometimes give confused signals? However, I do often feel like eating when I am not hungry. I think this can be due to habit, boredom, stress or cravings and so I am careful when I 'fancy' a snack. I try, as hard as I can, to have a drink rather than a snack. This not only feels me up a little bit; it warms me up, gives me something to do, distracts me and hopefully helps the wish for a snack to disappear. Of course, getting a drink does mean venturing into the kitchen, where the snacks are so it can be a very tricky to resist grabbing something to eat while I am there. I try very hard not to collect something 'in case I want it later' as I will always eat it.

Fruit and Vegetables

These are really good for us and an idea thing to snack on. Some fruit such as oranges and bananas even come in a case so that you do not need to wrap them up or prepare them in advance. It can be better to go for vegetables as they have lower sugar content and so a carrot could be a good portable option as long it is clean you do not need to peel it. Pears and apples can be great too as long as your teeth will allow you to bite straight into them. You could also consider having grapes, cherry tomatoes, berries or things like this which can be easily eaten with no preparation apart from a wash, which you can do beforehand. These might not be the most filling snacks though as they do contain a lot of water and the more sugary fruits might give us a sugar boost which could possibly be followed by a low. There are options below where you can combine fruit and vegetables with other things to make their energy last longer.

Nuts

Nuts are really healthy for us. Not only do they have lots of healthy fats they also have nutrients too. Walnuts even contain omega 3. Nuts are often available with oil and salt on and it is best, if you can to avoid these. Try to go for nuts which are roasted as these are easier to digest (Leong, 2013) but avoid the oils if you can. It may take a bit of getting used to but you can buy some nuts which have been roasted without oils and have salt or you can add your own salt if you cannot find them. However, do be careful with salt levels as we should not have too much, although we need some. Try to have a variety of different types of nuts as well as this means that you will get a bigger range of nutrients.

Many people are concerned about the fat in nuts and the calories. They are high in fat and calories but the fats are healthy ones and you should not need to eat lots of nuts to feel full or satiated. If you have salted ones you will tend to eat more, because the salt almost seems to have an addictive quality and makes you want eat more and more. If you have unsalted nuts then you will not get this compulsion to eat so many. Swapping from salted peanuts, for example, to unsalted can be hard. It could be better to start with a nut that you do not normally have salt and fat on like walnuts or Brazil nuts.

Try different types of nuts to see which you like the best or eat a variety to keep the snack interesting and more nutritious. Consider trying walnuts, pecan nuts, almonds, Brazil nuts, pistachio nuts, macadamia nuts, hazelnuts, peanuts and cashew nuts. You can even buy pieces of coconut to snack on these days. You should be able to find them all in your local supermarket or health food shop and they all have different flavours and so if you dislike one, there could be others that you do like.

Salted popcorn

You may be able to make this yourself using a saucepan or a popcorn machine but you can buy bags of popcorn ready-made, which are a lot more expensive but certainly more convenient. Many bags of popcorn will have sugar as well as other flavours and so it is best to avoid these but go for the ones that just have salt as they are much healthier. The popcorn itself is a good source of fibre and can be more filling than other snacks. Do watch the salt levels though, especially if you have high blood pressure or are sensitive to salt in any way. To make your own popcorn in a saucepan, start by making sure that you have a pan with a tight fitting lid. You want to also use a pan with a thick bottom and put it on a medium heat. Add 3 tablespoons of oil of your choice and warm the oil. You need the oil to be hot before putting in the popcorn and to test it you can drop in a few pieces and once it pops very carefully scoop it out and then add a thin layer of kernels to the bottom of the pan. Put on the lid and gently shake it as it pops. Once there are a few seconds between pops you can remove it from the heat, remove the lid and then tip into a bowl. Be careful in case any corn pops while you are doing this. Then you can add the flavouring of your choice such as salt or paprika.

Oatcakes and nut butter

This may not sound like the healthiest snack but as far as snacks go it can be pretty good. The oatcakes have a lot of fibre and although the oats are ground so they are not as fibrous as whole oats, they are still better for you than wheat crackers as they have more fibre and nutrients. The nut butter may sound bad, but nuts contain healthy fats and are much better than butter and alternatives. Do look for a nut butter without added sugar and check the salt content too. Some have added fats and it is best to buy one that is just the pureed nuts with nothing else added but these do tend to be more expensive. Butter is better than other fats, but is still high in calories, saturated fat and can have a negative influence on cholesterol. It is better than margarines and spreads because it is in its natural form and therefore free of harmful hydrogenated fats which spreads and margarines tend to have. Just make sure that you do not have too much butter and you can sandwich the biscuits together so that the butter is shared between two biscuits. You can also eat oatcakes with different types of nut butter, hummus, soft cheese and other toppings. Add fruit or salad vegetables to the top if you want to make them more exciting.

Veggies and hummus

A raw carrot can make a great snack. With its natural sweetness and crisp texture it can be lovely on its own as can some cucumber, celery, cherry tomatoes or sugar snap peas. However, many of us find things like this too boring and like to have them chopped up to dip into something to make a more appealing snack. This will take a while to prepare but you can buy vegetable sticks that are already cut if you do not want to and it is very easy to buy hummus these days. If you are not keen on hummus then you could opt for guacamole instead, although this tends to have a lot more added ingredients when you buy it in the supermarket compared to hummus. You could make your own though. It is easy to combine a drained tin of chickpeas with a few tablespoons of tahini, a splash of the chickpea water from the can and a clove or two of garlic in a food processor. You then just season to taste. Some people like to add olive oil or lemon juice or both. You can also add roasted vegetables or use beans instead of chickpeas to get different colours and flavours. Hummus is easy to make with a food processor but if you do not have one or do not have the time, then the shop made versions have the same ingredients as homemade so you probably gain very little health wise by making it yourself although you can make It to your own taste. With guacamole, you could be better off just mashing an avocado with a fork and adding some salt and other seasoning perhaps tomato and chilli as it is quicker and creates less washing up than using a food processor but check what your local supermarket has first as it could be pretty healthy anyway. Guacamole does tend to have more added ingredients than hummus though so you may prefer to keep things simpler and healthier by making your own.

Cheese

We have been lead to believe that cheese is really bad for us, but actually thinking is now changing. The fats in cheese are no longer seen to be as bad and the fact that it is alkaline means that it is good for your teeth as well. Just having a few small squares or thin slices can be really satisfying. Cheese is high in calories though and so you need to be careful how much you are having if you are trying to lose weight. Try just having a couple of 1cm cubed pieces or a thin slice (if you buy it sliced) and then wait for half an hour to see if you are still hungry.

Toast dipped in oil

If you have tasty wholemeal bread then it can be really delicious dipped in olive oil. Raw olive oil (i.e. unheated) has been shown to have positive heart benefits and there was no difference between the lighter refined oils and the extra virgin types (Silva et al. 2015) so you can pick the olive oil that you prefer the taste of. The bread dipped like this, can taste just like fried bread but with the oil being cold you get the extra health benefits from it, which can be lost when it is heated. A whole piece of toast may seem like a big snack but calorie wise it can compare to a grab bag of crisps or a chocolate muffin but it is much more filling and nutritious.

Fruit and cream or yogurt

This may sound rather too indulgent as well but there are good reasons for having the cream with the fruit. Fruit is obviously nutritious but it does not tend to fill us up for that long. The protein and fat in the cream or yogurt will fill us up though. Get full fat yoghurt as it fills you up for longer and do not get one with added flavourings as these always contain sugar. Yogurt has the added benefit of being particularly beneficial to our gut bacteria (Lara-Villoslada et al., 2007). If you are concerned about calories then just have more fruit and less yogurt rather than buying a lower fat version as these tend to be very sour and you may want to add sweeter fruits or even sugar or sweetener to them. Try different brands of yogurt to find one which has a pleasing flavour and consistency.

Toasted seeds

Seeds are great for fibre and they taste delicious when they are roasted as well as being easier to digest. Simply put some in a non-stick pan and heat until they start to brown. Then tip into a bowl and add a drizzle of olive oil and stir then add some salt to taste. Eat with a teaspoon as the oil makes them too difficult to handle! You can omit the oil and salt if you wish but they do add healthy fat and a delicious flavour as well.

Cereal

Many people use cereals as a snack and even buy cereal bars. We are lead to believe that these are healthy options but if you look at the ingredients you will see how much sugar they contain. However if you make your own cereals, using the simple recipes later in the book you will be able to have a sugar free version. The commercially available cereal bars though, really should be avoided as there are no versions available with no sugars.

Hard Boiled Egg

Keeping some hard boiled eggs in the fridge ready to snack on can be really handy. They are under 100 calories per egg and really filling. You could slice them into a sandwich if you are extra hungry or just eat them with a little salt or even some French mustard. If you prefer you could mash them with some mayonnaise, but do watch the mayonnaise as it usually has added sugar.

Olives

If you like olives then they can make a great snack. They are juicy and savoury and can be really satisfying. They contain healthy fats too. Try having different types of olives to get different flavours but be careful if you are buying stuffed ones to make sure that they are still healthy. If they are stuffed with cheese, for example, they will be a lot higher in calories which could be a problem if you are trying to lose weight. Olives come in oil or brine and you may prefer one to the other so it can be worth trying both types. The ones in oil will have more calories due to the oil but as the olives contain oil anyway it may not make that much difference.

Breakfasts

Breakfast is often a rushed affair with other jobs being done at the same time. There may be a dishwasher to unstack, washing to put on, lunch boxes to make, homework to do, emails to answer or all manner of things that seem to go on first thing in the morning. It is important though to have a healthy breakfast as a healthy start to the day can really help us to be healthier for the rest of the day. Therefore think about what you can have which is fairly quick to make but that will allow you to get a healthy start to the day. You may think that you do not have time to cook things, but you can just leave things slowly cooking while you get on with other jobs and so it does not have to take up that much time.

Below are a few ideas.

Omelette

An omelette takes very little time to cook and it is easy too. All you need to do is melt some butter in a pan, whisk up an egg and tip it into the pan, turning it over once the top has dried out. There are more sophisticated ways of making it and you will probably want to season the egg as you whisk it. However it takes minutes to make and there are lots of ways that you can make it more exciting. You can fill it will all sorts of things. If you have left over veg or potatoes from the evening before then these are perfect. You could slice some broccoli and microwave it until it is soft and pop that in it. Take a tin of sweetcorn and put some in or use some frozen peas and onion. Most people like a bit of cheese, but add some sliced tomatoes, mushrooms and finely sliced spinach and you a get a better flavour and more nutrients too. You can serve it with avocado or even a bit of lettuce to add more vegetables.

Mushrooms on toast

This is really simple to do with an easy hack. Most people peel mushrooms. This is not necessary and the skin has loads of nutrients. So just knock off any dirt and then slice them into a pan with a little oil. Leave them to cook and add some finely chopped garlic if you wish and pop some toast in the toaster and in a few minutes you will have a really tasty breakfast. You can add tomatoes and spinach into the pan for the last minute for added flavour and nutrition.

Tomato and avocado on toast

Avocado on toast is such a delicious thing to have but adding some tomatoes just adds another dimension to the flavour as well as adding in extra nutrients. All you have to do is mash the avocado with a fork and then butter it onto the toast and put the sliced tomatoes on top, which you can cook, but are lovely raw. You may want to add salt and pepper too. You can even top with mushrooms and a fried egg if you wish.

Granola

My sugar free granola recipe may take a bit of getting used to. It can be easier to not think of it as granola because granola is always sweet and this is not. This is the type of recipe that you make a big batch of in advance and then can eat it over a few weeks. I don't measure the ingredients and so it is more about proportions. You can add in any nuts and seeds. I tend to use a packet of flaked almonds as they are sweet and really delicious when toasted, pumpkin and sunflower seeds – a small bag of each because they are the only seeds one of my sons will eat and jumbo oats – probably about half a kilogram. All I do is take half a tablespoon of coconut oil and melt it in a saucepan. Then mix it with all of the other ingredients in a big bowl, transfer to two baking dishes and spread evenly. I then toast in the oven until they are starting to brown. Some people may prefer them more golden, but I like to keep them quite pale in colour so they are still crunchy but not too brown. You can try different seeds and nuts and also add flavourings such as orange zest & juice, cinnamon and vanilla.

The granola is great just with milk but to sweeten it up, fruit can be added. It is nice with blueberries, raspberries or sliced banana. It can be served with plain yogurt or cream too.

Fruit 'crumble'

This can be fairly quick to make and something which can be cooking while you are doing other things such as packing lunch boxes, sorting laundry, stacking the dishwasher or one of those other jobs we seem to squeeze into our mornings. Start with an apple per person and core it and chop it into small thin pieces. Leave the skin on and put in a pan with blueberries, blackberries or raspberries. Add a knob of butter or coconut oil and a generous splash of water and simmer gently. The juice will come out of the soft fruit and cook down to form a syrup. Once it is done, top with oats. You could use some of the granola mix if you have some ready-made or just use a handful of jumbo oats, some seeds and nuts of your choosing (they are even nicer if you toast them gently in a non-stick pan first). You can then add some milk, plain yogurt, cream or eat without. You can also top with some cinnamon or mixed spice if you wish.

Porridge

Porridge is quick to make and a lovely warm breakfast for a cold day. It can be cooked in the microwave which means that you can leave it cooking when you get on with other things. If you cook it with water then you can do this on the hob and leave it too, but if you cook with milk you will need to stir it. It still does not take that long and you get a lovely warm cereal which you can add all sorts of things to. I sometimes cook it with vanilla and then add blueberries. I top it with banana and almond butter. Or I cook it with cinnamon, ginger, seeds and crushed nuts in for a different taste and texture. You can try all sorts of combinations.

French toast

This can be something which sounds tricky but really isn't and you can flavour it in all sorts of ways as well. You will need bread, you can use any type at all. Then take an egg and crack it into a flat bowl big enough to put the bread in. Whisk the egg in the bowl until the yolk and white have combined and put in the bread. Turn it over so both sides get a chance to soak up egg. Then you cook in a frying pan with a little butter or oil. This is a great way to use up bread that is a bit dry as it will soak up more egg.

You can serve this with avocado, mushrooms and tomatoes, or have it on its own. You might like to add a little salt with the egg if you are having it as a savoury dish. However, many people like French toast as a sweet dish. If you want this then you could add vanilla or cinnamon in with the egg and then serve with fruit such as strawberries and banana. You can also top with plain yogurt.

Muesli

Making muesli is so easy. I have only recently discovered how to make a really easy batch and I wish I had tried it before! Most muesli starts with a base of oats. I do the same but sometimes buy rolled rye and rolled barley to mix with it. I get these from an independent shop but you can buy them online and from health food shops including big chains so they should not be too hard to find if you want to try them. I then add a mix of seeds and flaked almonds. You can add all sorts of different nuts too so sometimes I buy a bag of mixed nuts, crush them with my mortar and pestle and add those. Make a big batch and you can use it whenever you wish. Most muesli will have sultanas in. You can add these, but I prefer to use fresh fruit and so leave it without fruit when storing and just add some in when I eat it. Personally I enjoy this warm as well as cold, just popped into the microwave for a few minutes once I have added the milk, makes it more comforting on a cold morning.

Beans on toast

Beans on toast can be a great way to start the day. Although tinned beans may not be the healthiest thing, they have two types of vegetable in them so can be a step towards getting lots of vegetables in your day. They are so quick to heat up and can be done by the time the toast pops out of the toaster. To make beans even healthier you can make your own, but you may want to do these in advance and then keep them in the fridge to warm up when needed. I make mine with some finely chopped onion which I microwave with some water for a few minutes until soft. I then put this into a baking dish with borlotti beans, soy sauce and some salt and cover with passata and bake in the oven for an hour. I add Worcestershire sauce when it comes out as otherwise the flavour seems to disappear and I end up adding more. You can experiment with seasonings to adjust them to your taste.

Overnight Oats

These are quite trendy at the moment but can be a great way to have a breakfast waiting for you in the fridge. The idea is that you make it up the night before and pop in the fridge so it is all ready in the morning. You add milk to the oats and they will soften overnight so they will have the texture of porridge without you having to cook it. They will obviously be cold, which can also be great on a warm morning. Most people will add all sorts of things to the oats to add flavour, texture and nutrients. Nuts, seeds and fruit are often used to do this and it is wise to experiment with different combinations so that you can find a mix that suits you. You might also like to add spices such as cinnamon or ginger to add flavours. Try grating apple, pear or carrot into the bowl and then putting the oats and milk over them, they will not brown as the milk will protect them. When you come to serve it you may like to top it with seeds, flaked almonds or crushed nuts as well as berries and yogurt. There are lots of options and it is great fun to experiment to try out different things to see what you enjoy the most.

Leftovers

If you have any leftovers from the night before, then you can heat them up for breakfast. The idea of having a breakfast like this might be rather unusual but it can be far healthier than cereal and extremely quick to warm up. You might fry up some leftover vegetables with egg to make a scramble or pop the food in the microwave to warm it up and eat as it is. You could warm it up in the oven if you popped on the oven on rising and got the food in and then by the time you are showered and dressed it will be ready.

It can be good to start forgetting our food stereotypes and that we have to have certain foods for certain meals. It can be a lot healthier to ditch the cereal and bacon and have a completely different breakfast. This is not easy, we may have been brought up on a sweet breakfast for our whole lives (except perhaps having a fry-up on a Sunday) and sometimes the idea of having something cooked or savoury in the morning just does not appeal. However, we can change if we want to and try something new which could be the start of a whole new healthier lifestyle.

Lunches

In the UK we are a bit rubbish at weekday lunches. We might eat a sandwich at our desk or snack on a pasty while walking to the shop and follow it with a chocolate bar. We may buy a meal deal at a supermarket where we get tempted to not only have a sandwich but to add a sugary drink, chocolate bar and crisps to it because we are told it saves us money. We do not normally take the time to stop and enjoy our food and have something nutritious that will help us to get through the afternoon. On a weekend we might be better and sit down with the family and have something healthier but this tends to be the exception these days. There are plenty of healthy choices that we can make with regards to lunches and there are some below.

Salads

Some people just are not fans of salad and think that they are hard to make. The great news is that you can buy a healthy salad from a supermarket all prepared for you so you do not have to do the work. Also there are lots of different types of salad. Many of us will just think of lettuce and other leaves with a bit of dressing but there are so many types. You make salad based around couscous, pasta, rice or potato that you have left over, for example. You can add all sorts of dressing to give great flavour, although you do need to watch out for the sugar in them. Once you get into the habit of preparing a salad it does not take long. Chopping skills will soon get faster and you can use ingredients that are easy. For example, you can use tinned sweetcorn, beans and/or tuna which needs no chopping at all. You can buy small leaves which do not need any chopping either. You can just slice tomatoes and grapes in half to throw in the salad. You can slice or grate carrot on a grater which is quicker than making sticks. Pepper, radishes and cucumber take very little time to cube up. It need only take minutes to prepare a salad.

Veggies and hummus

Another lunch favourite is veggies and hummus and although it is in the snack section it is worth considering as a lunch dish. You can buy a tub of hummus easily and even get the veggie sticks pre-cut. However it does not take that much time to slice up some carrots, peppers, cucumber and/or celery to dip in. You can also use radish, sugar snap peas, cherry tomatoes and grapes which need little or no preparation. You can choose a different dip if you would rather, try to go for one that is low in sugar though. Hummus is good because it has protein and it counts towards your veggie count as chickpeas count towards your five a day. It also has garlic which is really good for our gut bacteria as well. If you like you can also dip in wholemeal pita bread, oatcakes or wholemeal toast strips.

Boiled eggs

These can be a convenient way to get a good protein lunch. You can cook them at home while having breakfast and quickly peel them and pop them in a lunch box or you can put them in with the shells on and peel them later. You might want to spread them through the day as they can be filling, having some as snacks (as suggested earlier) and some with lunch. Another idea is to chop them and add them to your salad or put them in a sandwich. If you are using mayonnaise or salad cream with the egg then check the ingredients and see which you think is healthiest by comparing the sugar levels in them. Try to include some vegetables or fruit with your lunch as well as the eggs though.

Cheese and oatcakes

Oatcakes are a great healthy alternative to bread as they tend to contain less sugar, less additives and are always whole grain but they will go soggy if you butter them in advance. You could take butter to put on them but an alternative is slices of cheese. You can put lettuce with them as well which goes really well with the cheese and adds a different sort of crunch. Alternatively a few cherry tomatoes on the side add some sweetness and contrast of flavour.

Healthy sandwiches

It is possible to make some really healthy sandwiches that taste really good. Adding in some salad can help to make them healthier and using a healthier bread. So use a whole grain bread to keep it healthy and then choose a couple of salad items to either put in it or on the side with it. It is good to try to avoid processed meats if you can and so go for chicken, cheese, egg, salmon or tuna as healthy protein fillings. Then go for some salad to go in such as lettuce, cucumber, tomato, grated carrot, sweetcorn or things like this. It may make a rather large sandwich so you may be better off filling a pitta or wrap with it all or making a separate side salad to go with your sandwich.

Falafel wraps

Falafels are a great source of protein and can be made easily or bought ready-made. They are mainly chickpeas and when you make them you can just put chickpeas in a food processor with a few tablespoons of whole grain flour and herbs and spices to flavour them. You can also add things like garlic or cooked onions which add extra flavours. You just have to shape the mix into balls and bake in the oven and you can pop them in the fridge when cool, for when you need them. However, you can buy them but these often contain added sugars. Choose a whole grain wrap and pop a couple in with some hummus and salad. You can use grated carrot, shredded lettuce and sliced cucumber or any salad items that you enjoy.

Mixed nuts

You do not have to have what you might think of as a 'proper meal'. Having a few mixed nuts can be filling and takes no preparation at all. Having some tomatoes or fruit with it will balance it out and you will have nothing to do but possibly peel it. This would be a quick and easy solution but healthier than a bag of crisps and a chocolate bar which might be an alternative that is equally as quick but far less healthy. Do be careful when buying nuts though as you can be tempted to buy mixed nuts that are roasted in unhealthy oils and heavily salted or mixed with dried fruit and chocolate. It is best to buy unroasted nuts and either eat them like this or roast them yourself with no oil.

Brown or black rice sushi

Sushi is getting really popular and so is often available to buy from supermarkets. Unfortunately white rice is not good for us but there are some places which have brown rice or black rice versions which are much better for us. Sushi often comes with healthy fish as well and possibly some vegetables too. There may not be very many vegetables though and so you might want to have some extras or some fruit to eat after it.

Granola

If you enjoy having cereal then why not have some granola for lunch? Using the recipe in the breakfasts section you can easily make a big batch of healthy granola and then have some of this for lunch. Do try to not have it for lunch and breakfast on the same day though as it is far healthier to have a variety of foods each day.

Leftovers

If you have any leftover food from the day before then you could use this as your lunch, if you have not already had it for breakfast! You will be able to warm it up in the microwave if you have access to one or it might be okay to eat cold, depending on what it is. You could even get into the habit of making too much food the day before so that you can always have something left for your lunch.

Evening meals

When the time comes to eat in the evening we can often feel tired and hungry before we start cooking and so it can be tempting to call for a food delivery. It is therefore important to make sure that we start preparing or cooking before we feel like this. For some people it can be best for them to prepare the meal as soon as they get in so that they do not sit down and get too comfortable so they do not feel like getting up again. For others they want to have a sit down and a drink before they start cooking. Consider which might suit you the best.

It can sometimes feel like cooking takes a really long time. Some meals do take a lot of preparation then a lot of cooking and need lots of fiddly sauces and ingredients and this can just be too much effort. It may be that you want something that just has ingredients that are easy to find or that are in your cupboard. Perhaps you want something that has just a few ingredients or just takes very little time to cook. There are recipes out there which can fulfil these criteria and there are also some tips below too.

Mominoes

This is a favourite in my family and a great substitute for a pizza take away. (The name came from a famous pizza delivery company combined with 'Mum' to make my healthy version!) Just use wholemeal bread as the pizza base and toast it on one side under the grill. Then turn it over and add sliced tomato (or spread on some tomato paste or passata) and top with some grated cheese and grill. You can enhance the flavour by putting dried herbs such as oregano or basil on the tomato. If you have a bit more time then you can add extra veg. I tend to fry up some sliced onions, peppers and mushrooms and put them under the cheese to add extra nutrients and flavour. If you do not eat bread then you can use a cooked omelette as a base instead. You can eat together with some salad if you do not have the other vegetables.

Fish and Chips

It is really easy to go to the chip shop or to put some frozen fish in the oven and some chips in the deep fat fryer, but there are healthy alternatives which do not have to take that much longer. Making your own chips can be very simple. I always use potatoes with good skins and leave the skin on and cut them into thick wedges for speed. If I want to be even healthier I use sweet potatoes instead of white potatoes. I boil them for five minutes, but you could microwave them after cutting them for the same amount of time. Then I brush them with olive oil and cook in the oven for about 45 minutes. Cook the fish in the oven with them but cook some plain salmon or other oily fish if you like it or some white fish. You can flavour them with herbs or spices or make a tomato salsa to eat with them from a shallot fried with about half a dozen cherry plum tomatoes and salt. Cook some vegetables to go with the dish as well, peas is an obvious choice but why not put some mangetout, broccoli, carrots or other veg with it too. You could microwave a bag of mixed vegetables for speed. You will end up with a meal that has less fat and less sugar but still gives you a tasty treat and does not take ages to cook. It can be very satisfying to take a few minutes to prepare a meal and then pop it in the oven and you can relax or catch up with other jobs while it cooks.

Rice Salad

This is a really easy dish to make, can be served hot or cold and can be made in advance. You will need to start by cooking the brown rice. I always soak rice overnight and wash it a lot to ensure that it does not have too much arsenic in it (Moseley, 2017), but you can just follow the packet instructions or for speed buy a packet of precooked brown rice.

I tend to use onions, pepper, peas and carrots in my rice salad, but you can use whatever you wish. I chop them really small and then cook them in a little water and oil in a pan until they are soft. They could be microwaved or you could cook them in with the rice. Once they are all cooked, I mix them together adding a crumbled stock cube or some stock powder and a teaspoon of turmeric. You can add whatever flavourings you wish but I find these add the colour and seasoning that I like.

Vegetable Stew

This is such an easy thing to make and can take little preparation if you cheat as well. You can add any vegetables that you like and then make the gravy to suit you. I tend to always have some key ingredients which add flavour and then pop in anything extra that I have. So I always use a chopped onion, you could use the frozen pre chopped onions. Then I add a few carrots, you do not need to peel carrots, just make sure they are clean, cut off top and bottom and dice them. I also add frozen peas and sweetcorn and sometimes frozen broad beans or edamame beans. I then put in either new potatoes which I leave the skins on and dice or sweet potato which are healthier. I put in some sort of greens perhaps sprouts (you could use frozen) or cabbage which you can buy already chopped up. Then I either put in orange lentils which I just wash first, or tinned mixed beans but you could use other types of lentils, beans or chickpeas if you prefer. I cover all with water and bring the pan to the boil and leave it to simmer for ten minutes while I get on with other jobs and then check to see if the vegetables are cooked. Once they are cooked I add stock cubes, soya sauce and Worcestershire sauce. These do have sugar in but I do not use much and have not yet found a sugar free version and I do not use very much. I tend to serve this over some wholemeal couscous for speed (the couscous can even be tipped into the stew for the last five minutes to hydrate) or with some crusty wholemeal bread. It would be lovely with homemade wholemeal dumplings or with wholemeal cheese scones on the side.

Stir Fry

This is a really easy meal to cook and full of vegetables. You can serve it with brown rice or whole wheat noodles. If you do not like chopping vegetables then you can buy bags of pre prepared stir fry vegetables. However, chopping an onion, pepper, mushrooms, broccoli, pak choi and things like that does not take long. It is best to start by softening the onion in a pan with some olive oil and splash of water before adding in the other vegetables. You can also add in chicken, tofu or other protein sources such as chickpeas or nuts to make it a balanced meal. Marinated tofu tends to have a lot of sugar added so marinate your own with sugar free soy sauce or buy smoked tofu instead if you like the flavour. Use a sugar free soya sauce to flavour it. You can buy stir fry sauces but these can be very sugary so check the label first and decide whether it is something that you want to eat.

Easy Peasy Pasta

Pasta is really easy to cook and you can buy stir in sauces or pesto to put on it so that you can get a meal very easily. There are ways that you can easily make your pasta meal healthier. Firstly weigh out 30-50g wholemeal pasta per person depending on how hungry they are. Then dice a whole onion into rough squares and add it in. You can use frozen pre-chopped onion if you wish. Also add in a diced red pepper, some diced mushrooms and a diced courgette. The amount of veg you use depends on how many people are eating the meal. I tend to do half of each vegetable per person. Then put all these veg in with the pasta and cook it until the pasta is done. I check it by eating a bit after about ten minutes. Once the pasta is cooked the vegetables will be as well so drain them all off and then put on your sauce. The healthiest choices would be a sugar-free pesto or passata. I tend to also add herbs such as dried oregano or basil as well as a little salt if needed. Then simmer the sauce to warm it up and add in a handful of finely shredded spinach per person. Once the spinach has wilted it is cooked. If you prefer you can fry the onions until soft then add the pepper, mushrooms and courgette and fry those and once they are cooked put on the sauce and add the spinach. The first method obviously uses just one pan so is easier but the peppers particularly have a very different flavour when they are fried rather than boiled, so this depends on your taste as well. Also boiling vegetables can leach out a lot of the vitamin C into the cooking water, which does not happen with frying, but as long as we have some raw fruit or vegetables in our diet it is unlikely that we will be low in vitamin C anyway.

Baked Potato and Beans

This is a surprisingly easy meal to make and just takes a little bit of preparation and can be left to cook in the oven. Firstly you need to preheat the oven to 200 degrees and scrub the sweet potatoes and cut out any bad bits and stab the skin in several places. Put in the microwave for five minutes. Meanwhile chop up an onion into small cubes and put into a microwavable dish. Once the potatoes come out of the microwave, pop in the onion for a couple of minutes covering with some water first. Put the potatoes onto an oven tray and put in the oven. Then put the onions into an oven dish. Drain a tin of haricot (or borlotti) beans and put in the dish too. Then cover with passata. Add a pinch of salt and stir and put in the oven too. Then you can just leave everything to cook for an hour. When it is ready, stir some Worcestershire sauce into the bean mixture and slice the potatoes in half and cover with the beans.

Roast Dinner

A roast dinner can take a lot of time to prepare, so it is not a quick meal but many people will make them regularly and there are lots of ways that you can make it healthier without making major changes. The meat may be considered by some to be the unhealthiest due to the saturated fats but if you just have a small amount then this could be fine for you. It can be the marinades, sauces and gravies that are more of a problem so have a think about what you are using and whether you can make it healthier, perhaps by making your own or just flavouring with a rub of spices. Roasted potatoes also need to be eaten with caution. Consider whether the oil you are using is safe to cook at a high temperature in the oven as some are unstable and unhealthy at high temperatures. Also note that potatoes are very easily broken down into sugar so having less of them could be sensible. Leaving on the skins and cooking in less oil will be a healthier option. You could also replace some potatoes with less sugary vegetables such as parsnips, sweet potatoes, squash and carrots. Boiled vegetables are often served with a roast. If you are having these then do a big variety of different vegetables being sure to add in some greens in the form of cabbage, sprouts or broccoli. If you do not have enough saucepans then cook vegetables together in one pan.

Leftover Bake

This is a great recipe for using up any leftover vegetables that you may have, whether cooked or uncooked. You will need 30g whole wheat macaroni per person, leeks or onions and other selected vegetables. Start by cooking the macaroni with any vegetables you have that need cooking, things like broccoli, cauliflower, carrots, sweet potatoes work well. Then finely chop the onions or leeks. About one onion or leek between two people will be enough for flavour. Fry the leek or onion in a splash of water and butter and once soft add about 25g extra butter and melt. Then stir in 1 tablespoon whole grain plain flour and stir. Then add two heaped teaspoons of French mustard and stir. Then slowly add milk until you get a runny sauce. Bring to the boil and then add salt, pepper and a handful of grated cheese and cook gently until the cheese has melted. Your pasta and vegetables should be cooked by now so test them to see. Once cooked, add to a baking dish with any pre-cooked leftovers you may have such as potatoes, squash, greens or anything else. You can also add tinned sweetcorn and finely chopped spinach. Pour the sauce over the vegetables and then top with a layer of grated cheese and bake in a moderate oven for 45 minutes or until the sauce is bubbling and the top is starting to brown.

Couscous and Vegetables

Couscous is so easy to cook it is a great way to prepare a really fast meal. You can add salad vegetables or some cooked vegetables with beans or chickpeas to it to make a balanced meal. You can also serve it alongside meat or fish.

The couscous will not need cooking but just hydrating. This is easily done by adding boiling water as per the instructions on the packet. It can be much tastier though if you use stock. You can easily do this by using a stock cube in the water.

You can add all sorts of vegetables. For a salad you can add spring onions, tomatoes, cucumber, pepper and radish and for a warm dish fry up some onions, peppers, mushrooms and spinach to make a lovely dish. You can easily use any vegetables that you have available.

Curry and Rice

This might seem like a really hard meal to cook but it can actually be very easy. If you make it at home you can include lots of vegetables and use wholegrain rice and spices that you enjoy. Some people would buy a spice blend or curry powder, some would buy a curry paste and others would make their own blend. Some pastes will have sugar in so it can be better to use a curry powder and you can use yogurt or coconut cream or milk to make the sauce. I make a vegetarian curry but you could add some chicken if you wished to.

I start by putting on the rice to cook according to the packet instructions. Then I peel sweet potatoes and put them onto boil in a small saucepan just covered with water. Then in a large frying pan cook finely chopped onion in a tablespoon of oil with some water and once it is soft add some garlic and spices. I use a teaspoon each of turmeric, cumin and coriander (and would also add some grated fresh ginger if my children would eat it!) but you can use what you like and most people would probably want chilli or cayenne pepper but I have to make it child friendly so with no heat. I cook this for a minute and then add frozen peas and pour in tinned coconut cream and a teaspoon of lemon juice (it can be the concentrated type from a bottle). I add a stock cube or stock powder at this stage and then a few handfuls of finely shredded spinach (and would add in a tin of drained chickpeas if my son would eat them). Once the sweet potato is cooked I add that in with the cooking water as well so that the sauce is runnier and you get the goodness from the water in the dish.

You can add in any vegetables that you have; squash, cauliflower and butter beans work well in this sort of curry but throw in any leftovers you need to use or any vegetables that need using up. You can add meat, paneer or prawns too, but you would need to make sure that it was well cooked in the pan just after cooking the onions.

Puddings

We all know that puddings are not healthy but giving them up can be really hard particularly if we are in the habit of having them daily. It may be that you just serve them as a treat when you have guests or it is a special occasion. Now for some people having the odd pudding is okay, they can have one and then go without for a long time. However, I find that once I start having some sugar I want more and more things with sugar in. I start thinking that it is okay for me to have it, start craving sweet things and find that I start eating lots of sugary foods and put on lots of weight and make poor decisions when making food choices. I therefore avoid sugar as much as I can and do not have puddings at home, when I am out or when I am visiting others unless it is fruit. However, there are things that you can replace puddings with which are free of added or refined sugars which could help you get used to not having pudding.

Coffee

Having a milky coffee after a meal, particularly if it is a cappuccino or latte can really help you to feel like you have had a pudding. It can be filling and I find milky coffee quite sweet without needing to add sugar or sweetener. Obviously I am not used to having things that sweet and I used to have sugar in coffee but am now very used to it without and can taste the natural sweetness in the coffee and the milk. If it is hot weather and you have a blender you can make a coffee milkshake from milk, a shot of coffee and ice.

Cheese

Having a cheeseboard is often offered as an alternative to pudding in restaurants or after pudding. It can be a great to end a meal without having to have a pudding. You can put fruit with it; pear, apples and grapes can all go well with different cheeses. Having a selection can be fun as well. Do make sure though, that you be careful about the crackers that you choose to go with the cheese. Many crackers are made of refined white flour and have unhealthy fats in them. There are some wholemeal crackers available as well as oatcakes but you will even need to check these carefully as they could have added sugar.

Fruit

This may sound boring but it really does not have to be. There are so many different fruits that you can choose from and you can serve them in lots of different ways and combinations. You can have yogurt or cream with them, have one type of fruit or a fruit salad. Making a fruit crumble is really easy as well. You can just put the granola on top of cooked fruit or make a crumble from whole grain flour, butter, oats and spices (for example rub 75g butter into 250g wholemeal flour and 50g oats). If I have cinnamon in the fruit I add a teaspoon of mixed spice into the crumble mix otherwise I add the cinnamon into the topping. However with some fruits vanilla works better, for example with raspberries or peaches, whereas cinnamon is lovely with apple. As long as the fruit is naturally sweet you should not need any sugar. You may find that it takes time to get used to having this sort of thing without sugar but you can slowly reduce the sugar you add in or you can use a sweetener instead but beware that some of these have bad effects on our gut bacteria. Try to use a minimum amount and reduce it too so that you do not get used to things having such a sweet taste.

Coffee mousse

This probably sounds terribly wicked but there are two ways of making it which will minimise the sugar. I simply use a tub of mascarpone cheese and then add in some very concentrated coffee.

You do need to be careful that the coffee is not too hot or else it separates the cheese and goes greasy. Make a very strong shot of coffee, boil it down in a saucepan so it is very concentrated (about a tablespoon) and add that to the cheese once it is cool to make a coffee mousse. If you do not mind instant coffee then you can just dissolve as much as you can in a tablespoon of boiling water and then stir that in once it cools. You will always need to set the mousse in the fridge.

Summer Pudding

This is traditionally made with white bread and sugar but it can easily be made with wholemeal bread and unsweetened fruit. You can choose any soft fruits such as strawberries, raspberries, currants, blueberries and blackberries. It is good to use sweet fruits if you have a sweet tooth, although it will be cheaper if you use frozen fruit. Cook the fruits slightly to soften them and let out some juices and you can add vanilla which adds sweetness and flavour at this point. You will need a basin which you line with the bread. Usually you remove the crusts from the bread as you want the bread to absorb the juices from the fruit. Do not waste the crusts; you can use them to make breadcrumbs. You need to grease the basin with oil or butter and line with cling film. Then press the bread onto all the edges and base of the basin, so the amount that you need will depend on the size of the basin you use. Fill the centre with the fruit and then top with more bread. The aim is to have a layer of bread all around the fruit. Then wrap the cling film over the top and put it in the fridge overnight to cool, before removing the cling film and tipping onto a plate an serving with cream or yogurt.

Scones

Scones are easy to make and they come out the same way whether you use wholemeal or white flour and whether or not you include sugar. This means they can be made as great treat without having the sugar in them and with having the whole grain flour. They are very simple to make just rub 50g butter into 200g self-raising wholemeal flour (or plain flour with 4 tsp baking powder) until it forms breadcrumbs then add 150ml milk. You can use all sorts of flours such as wheat, spelt, buckwheat or whatever type you enjoy or can tolerate. I find that wholegrain spelt flour is lighter when baking compared to wheat so tend to use this if I have it. The milk you use can also vary, as you may prefer a plant based milk, and this will work fine. However, if use different grains and or milk, you may need different amount of milk. Therefore add it slowly until the mixture just holds together.

You can add flavours into them or just have them plain and top with flavoured items. For example you can add vanilla to the scone mix and then top with strawberries and cream. You can add cinnamon and apple to the scones before baking and then top with almond butter. Of course you can add cheese and herbs, sundried tomatoes, cooked onion or things like this to make a delicious savoury version to accompany stews or to just eat with butter.

Carrot Cake

It can be tempting to think that a carrot cake is always healthy because it has vegetables in it. Sadly this is not the case as it also normally has sugar and possibly unhealthy fats in it as well. However, it is possible to make your own healthier version. Cakes still have a lot of fat in and are high in calories but this can be used for a rare treat. You will just need to grate 150g carrots and one sweet eating apple and mash two ripe bananas with a fork. Then put 280g self-raising wholemeal flour in a bowl with 1 tsp baking powder and 1 tsp mixed spice. Beat 3 eggs and add in the bowl with the carrot, banana, 60g sultanas and 170ml light olive oil or melted butter. Mix it all together and put in a lined cake tin and bake at 180 degrees for 50-60 minutes until cooked. If you want to add icing then use cream cheese and add in some vanilla or lemon juice for flavour. If you need it to be sweeter then you could use a little honey. You can slice it through the middle and put some icing in it or just spread on the top and decorate with walnut halves.

Strawberry Milkshake

This is a great recipe for the summer as it is best when the strawberries are really ripe and sweet. It is easy to make with a blender, but you can make it without if you have a metal sieve. You just need to add 10 strawberries to a pint of milk and then blend. However, if you push the strawberries through a sieve it will remove the seeds and then you can just stir the juice into the milk or use a balloon whisk to make it frothy. This seedless version might be preferred by children anyway. You can use the juice to pour over ice cream or yogurt rather than putting it into a milkshake if you wish. It will take time to sieve the fruit but you may find that children want to help with this as it can be fun.

Ice-cream

This is not normal ice-cream but a fruit ice-cream. The main base is bananas as they freeze really well. You will need a blender or food processor for this recipe. You need to slice up some ripe bananas and put them in the freezer. Once they are frozen solid you blend them with yogurt or cream to make your ice cream. You can eat right away or freeze again, although once refrozen it will be really hard. You can add different fruits, such as strawberries or flavours such as vanilla but you will always need the banana to get the right texture.

Go without

Of course, it might just be best to go without pudding altogether. If you are trying to reduce how much you eat, avoid having so much sugar and generally be healthier than avoiding puddings can be a good way to go about it. Having one occasionally or when you have guests may be a nice treat, but having something every day can be a habit which we should perhaps not be trying to get into.

All About Vegetables

Many people do not eat enough vegetables but they do not like them and so tend to avoid them. This could be from being put off them as children after having bitter soggy cabbage, spongy slimy mushrooms and dry butter beans. However, there are so many vegetables and they can be prepared and cooked in so many different ways that it is worth taking a look through this list to see if there are any that you would like to try. Most people have some foods that they do not like but not eating any vegetables means that you are eliminating a very healthy selection of foods. Vegetables vary a lot in taste and texture and so it is worth giving them a go.

Carrots

Carrots and very versatile and often liked by people because they are sweet. They are never bitter and have a texture that can vary depending on whether served raw or cooked. They are easy to prepare and do not even need to be peeled, although always wash a vegetable if you are not peeling it and remove any blemishes from the skin. They can be eaten raw, perhaps grated in salads and sandwiches or cut into batons to scoop up dip. If you find cutting batons too time consuming, you can buy carrots already cut into batons, which will be expensive but save you time. Although, like all fruit and vegetables, they are good source of vitamin C when raw, they can be better for you when cooked. Cooking can cause the water soluble vitamin C to leach out into the cooking water but if you eat raw fruit and vegetable or a great deal of them you will not be deficient anyway. Carrots contain beta-carotene which is much easier for the body to extract when cooked (Imsic et al., 2010).The more you cook it; the more you can get out which means that a carrot soup has more in than plain boiled carrots. Carrots can also be roasted, which caramelises them and makes them taste even sweeter. They are a great addition to soups as they add an overall sweet taste.

Peas

Peas are so easy because you can buy them podded and ready to cook. You can buy them fresh in season and frozen all of the year round. They have a sweet flavour and there are different types which have slightly different flavours and textures. You can buy peas dried as well and soak them and then boil them to make mushy peas or you can buy these in a tin but they tend to have added sugar if you buy them this way. Peas are such an easy addition to any meal as you can use the fresh ones raw in salad or heat them up by boiling, steaming or microwaving to produce a very quick side vegetable. They can be easily stored in the freezer to use in any dish, such as adding to stews, stir fries, curries, sweet and sour or with mash.

Cabbage

Cabbage is a vegetable that many people do not like having had very bitter varieties as children and having them boiled until they were soggy. However, there are many different types of cabbage with different flavours and many different ways of cooking them. Firstly if you are going to boil cabbage make sure that it is well drained so that it is not soggy. Tossing it around in the strainer should get rid of any excess water. You can also use cabbage in stir-fry which can change the texture.

Consider what type of cabbage you are using as they can taste very different. The dark cabbages such as cavalo nero and kale have more of a flavour whereas lighter cabbages such as spring greens and white cabbage are much sweeter. Sprouts can be lovely if they are well cooked. You can buy them frozen but these tend not to cook well - being hard in the centre and soggy on the outside. If you cook fresh sprouts you can stop this happening by cutting them in half and then only cooking them for five minutes. However, you may think that sprouts are too difficult to prepare but some supermarkets now sell ready prepared sprouts which are much easier. They will be more expensive but if you can afford it and want to save time, they can be a good alternative.

Cabbage can also be eaten raw in coleslaw. Sweeter varieties such as white and red cabbage tend to be used. These are finely shredded and added to shredded onions and carrots and served with mayonnaise. They are very easy to make if you have a food processor and you can buy them already made. Do be careful with buying them premade as they can often have a lot of added sugar as well as other additives.

Broccoli and Cauliflower

Both of these often have bad memories from childhood of being cooked until they were soggy or served in a split and under seasoned cheese sauce. There are ways to cook them so that they do not go soggy though. If you are boiling them make sure that you use even sized florets, then use a blunt knife to poke through the stems every couple of minutes to see if they feel soft. As they start to soften feel more often until they are cooked to your liking. Some people prefer to eat them raw with dips.

Preparing them is very easy which is a great advantage of these. You hardly need a knife as you can rip them apart. You can buy them frozen for convenience but it is very difficult to cook them well if you do this as they can easily go soggy.

Normally these two would be cooked in the same way, just boiled. However, they can be roasted. These days it is becoming fashionable to add spices and then roast them until they start to crisp. You can use plain spices such as salt and pepper or have something more exotic if you like it. You could even just very thinly slice them and roast them in the oven with some cheese on the top. They can also be used in a curry or stir fry but it can be wise to cook them a little first so they are not hard, a few minutes blanched in boiling water if they are small piece or a few minutes in the microwave should be enough. If you get the long stemmed versions then these can work well griddled as well as steamed.

Onions

We may have experienced onions either pickled or on burgers but they are very versatile and can be used in lots of different dishes. They are very good for the gut bacteria so having lots can be really good for you. Some people do find that they can cause them to get wind but this can be helped by making sure that they are cooked until soft.

Spring onions can be handy as they can be really easily prepared and chopped into salads or any other dish that you are cooking. Long, thin shallots can be great if you do not have much time for preparation. You just have to peel them and split them longwise and then you can shred or cube them really quickly or easily.

Onions are really good for our gut bacteria and they add great flavour to many different dishes. Whether you put them in a curry, stew or soup or fry them to go on a burger or shred them to go with cheese in sandwiches or in coleslaw; they are certainly very versatile. It is worth trying different types of onions if you do not like some. This is because they have different flavours and textures. You will also find that different ways of preparing and cooking them will change the flavour so the strength you get when raw is not so apparent once cooked and if cooked for a long time they will caramelise and go very sweet.

Marrow, courgette and squash

You may remember having roasted marrow as a child with your roast dinner. These were peeled, seeds scooped out and cut into semi-circular pieces and roasted. They went all soft and squashy. These days it is much more common to see courgettes and other sorts of squash in the shops than marrow. Courgettes are rather like a baby marrow but their skins are softer so can be eaten and they do not need seeds removing. They can be cooked in a similar way by roasting if you like this method. They cook fairly quickly so can be a great addition to stir-fries, pasta sauces and things like this. They are also great mixed with aubergine, peppers and onions and roasted up. Finely chopped, this roasted vegetable mix can be used as a topping for pizza, in toasties with cheese or as a tasty filling for a tart.

Squashes are also part of the same family, but tend to be used to make soups or are roasted. There are lots of different types such as pumpkins, acorn squash and butternut squash. These tend to have orange flesh and very hard skin. Some people chop, remove the seeds and roast together with the skin to save effort, but the skin can be tough so you may prefer to remove it. Some squashes have a slightly bitter flesh and so may benefit from being added to other sweeter ingredients, but butternut squash tends to be sweeter and therefore does not need other things adding to it.

Squashes are sometimes baked in the oven stuffed with different fillings. This can be a good way to serve many vegetables if you feel that they need more flavour or excitement. You can stuff them with other vegetables such as onions and tomatoes and top with cheese or with flavoured mince or even couscous. There are lots of options that you can choose from.

Parsnip, Swede and Turnips

These root vegetables could be items that we remember for our childhood. They might have been boiled and mashed or served roasted. Some people may have memories of disliking them and others may like them. It can be worth revisiting them to see whether you still have the same feelings about them.

You can be more inventive than perhaps you once were as well. Although they can be added to soups and stews, roasting them can also make for an interesting and tasty alternative. Mashing them and eating instead of mashed potato can be a healthier option and they can be used as mash to top pies such as shepherd's pie and cottage pie to provide more vegetable portions.

They are not eaten raw and skins are usually removed so you will have to spend some time preparing them. However if you buy larger ones, you will not have as many to peel and thicker parsnips are easier to peel than thinner ones.

Another similar vegetable you could consider using is a Jerusalem artichoke. They are in season for a very limited amount of time and are very knobbly so peeling can be tricky. However, if you scrub them and roast them you may find that you will enjoy it without the skin being removed.

Tomatoes

Tomatoes may seem rather old fashioned and boring but they are actually very versatile and very good for us. They are often used in salads, but many people say that they do not taste as good as they used to. This can all depend on the type of tomato that you buy and where you buy them from. It can be tempting to think that the brightest red will be the tastiest. However, growers realise that buyers tend to want the reddest fruit and so grow the varieties that are a bright colour but also have good shelf life and this can mean that taste is sacrificed. This means that it is worth trying a combination of different varieties to see whether you can find one that tastes better. You will find that if you buy them in season, then the taste is likely to be better too. Local farmers markets may stock better tasting tomatoes or you could have a go at growing them yourself.

Tomatoes have a mix of nutrients but one of the most interesting is lycopene which is an antioxidant and good for the heart. It is more easily absorbed by the body if the tomato is cooked so tomato puree is better than fresh tomatoes with regards to the available lycopene in it. It can be used to intensely flavour a number of different dishes such as tomato based curries and be used as a topping on a pizza base.

Mushrooms

Some people, especially children struggle with the texture of mushrooms. They are very versatile and add a depth of flavour to food which is hard to replicate in any other way. They can be eaten raw (only good when really fresh!) or cooked in many ways. They are very quick to prepare as well, you do not need to do much but knock off the dirt and trim the stalk. Some people peel them as well, but this is optional. Skin can sometimes be tough especially if you bake, roast or fry the mushrooms whole, so the texture may be more desirable without it.

Mushrooms can be used to flavour stews, work well in curries, pasta sauces and stir fries or are lovely fried in some olive oil on toast, perhaps with garlic, onion or herbs such as sage added to give more flavour.

There are many different types of mushroom and these vary in flavour and texture which means that it can be worth trying a variety of them, particularly if there are some that you are not keen on. Dried mushrooms can be very much dearer but they add a much more intense flavour to dishes and so can be used sparingly or on special occasions.

Lettuce

Lettuce may seem like a very dull ingredient but it can actually add sweetness, pepperiness and crunch to many dishes. It is extremely easy to prepare as you can buy bags of leaves washed and ready to eat or you can just roughly chop up whole lettuces. It is wise to try out all sorts of different leaves to see which ones you like. Some people prefer the more peppery and bitter leaves to add a depth of flavour such as rocket and others like sweeter lettuce like romaine hearts. It is worth finding out what you like and do not like as you may be put off by lettuce you do not like but with so many different leaves to choose from you should be able to find one that you like.

Although a few people do bake lettuce it is usually served raw making it something really quick to prepare for eating. It can form the base of a salad but also be put in pitas, wraps and sandwiches. It is good to eat lots of leafy greens and the darker green the better so having lettuce can really be healthy for you.

Cucumber

Cucumber is often just popped in a salad but it can be used for so many things. It is easy to prepare by just slicing or cubing. It can even be made into scoop shapes or batons for serving with dips. Although the skin is good for us, some people find it difficult to digest and if this is the case it can be removed.

Cucumber goes well in sandwiches too particularly with tuna and salmon but also works with any salad or cheese as well. It may not taste that strong but not only adds a crunch but also adds to how many vegetables you are eating in a day, which can only be good for you.

Spinach

Spinach is a really versatile vegetable which can be added into all sorts of dishes. Leafy greens are really nutritious and although spinach is not as high in iron as it was first thought, it is still a good source. Spinach just needs to be washed and you can shred it if you wish but it is not necessary. It is extremely simple to cook, if you decide to cook it, but it can also be eaten raw. The young leaves tend to be sweeter and so are better for those that do not like bitter greens and are also good for eating raw.

You can pop spinach into salads in the same way that you would do with lettuce. You can also put them into all sorts of different cooked dishes. It goes well with tomato pasta dishes including lasagne, stir fries, curries and stews and can also be chopped into omelettes. It can even just be wilted and served as a side. Some people like to serve it with lemon juice but this will enhance the bitterness so if you find it too bitter then serve creamed instead.

Celery

Celery tends to be loved or hated by people. The stringiness can be unappealing and sometimes the flavour as well. If you buy it in season though, it tends to be less stringy and sweeter in flavour. You can also peel the stringy bits with a vegetable peeler, which tend to be on the outside of the larger and tougher stalks. It can be eaten raw in salads, used for dips or chopped into a mixed salad or even filled with nut butter or soft cheese. It can also be cooked and is often used as a base for stews. If you do not like it raw or cooked, then consider trying it the other way as you could find that you do like it this way.

When you are cooking celery think about the texture. You may have had it in stews where it could have gone really soggy. You may be able to find better ways to cook it where it is soft but not soggy. It can work in stir fries, for example. The leafy tops can be used as an alternative to lettuce or other leaves in a salad.

Sweetcorn

Sweetcorn comes in many forms, in a tin, frozen or fresh on the cob. There are different ways to eat it and the sweetness and subtle crunch can lift many dishes. Sweetcorn does need to be cooked and when you buy it tinned or frozen it already has been. However, if you buy it fresh on the cob you will need to cook it. You can simply boil it, but some people choose to cook it on the barbecue or griddle. It can be tricky to eat when on the cob, but you can buy small forks to hold the cobs with so that you do not burn your hands on it when trying to eat it. It can be delicious served with some butter.

Tinned sweetcorn tends to be sweeter than frozen and so this may affect how you use it. It is also generally more expensive. As it is ready to eat, it can be a great addition to salads. Some varieties will have sugar and salt added so check the tin before you buy to see whether you are happy with what it contains. Frozen sweetcorn will need defrosting, which you can do in the microwave or as you cook it and it goes really well in stews, with spicy Mexican beans or in stir fries. Not many vegetables are yellow and so it can add a lovely colour as well as a great flavour.

Peppers

Peppers are generally available in red, yellow, orange and green colours. These all have slightly different flavours, with the green perhaps having a slight bitterness and the red being sweeter. This is because the green peppers are unripe so not so sweet. They are really versatile and their bright colours can make dishes look really vibrant and attractive. They can be eaten raw, perhaps diced into salads or cut into strips and put into wraps or used with dips.

Peppers are also lovely cooked and can add a great base for many dishes. They are great in a stir fry, pasta sauce or savoury rice. They are easy to prepare as you just need to wash, and remove the stalk and seeds and you can chop in any way you wish. If you use a mixture of colours you can get really pretty dishes. Cubed peppers look great mixed in with rice or couscous salads either raw or chopped.

Avocado

Avocado is a "cool" vegetable at the moment. This is probably due to all of the health benefits, such as healthy fats. It is worth noting that it can be high in calories though, so you need to be careful how much you have and how often, if you are trying to cut down. It is extremely versatile as well, but it does oxidise and goes brown, very quickly, like fruit does. Therefore, you need to delay cutting it until just before you want to use it or you need to use lemon with it.

Avocado can be cut and mixed in with salad, but there are other ways that you can use it as well. It is delicious mashed with salt and spread on toast (particularly if topped with tomatoes and mushrooms!) or used as a dip. Some people bake avocado, but this completely changes the flavour and I think that it is an acquired taste.

Avocado is expensive and sometimes when you buy an avocado it can be overripe and stringy or black inside. I always buy 'ripe and ready to eat' avocado in packaging. This means that it cannot get bruised from people feeling it to see if it is ripe and it seems to be much better quality I pay a bit more for these but very rarely have any waste compared to cheaper ones which I waste far more often and consider are a 'false economy'. This may vary between supermarkets though so try different ones and see which you think give you the best value for money.

Summary

I hope that you now have enough information to encourage you to make some changes to your lifestyle. Hopefully you will now have a selection of tips that you want to try out that you can use to improve your health. Most of us know that there are ways that we can improve our health but think that it will not be easy to make those changes. Hopefully you will now have enough information that you will be able to use to make changes which will allow the transition to a healthier lifestyle to be a lot easier.

You may find it easier if you make a list of the changes that you want to make and tick off each one as you do it. It may be a slow process and this is fine. You need to make the changes at a pace that will suit you and your lifestyle. Do not put pressure on yourself to be 'perfect'. No one is perfect or eats perfectly all of the time and if we find that we are felling this way we could get stressed and this will not be healthy for us. So be kind to yourself and patient and try to enjoy the changes that you are making and hopefully you will feel the benefits too, with improvements to your health.

Good luck and I hope that this book will help you to make some steps in the right direction so that you can have a healthier lifestyle and therefore live a longer life and stay healthier while you are doing so.

References

Biessel, G. J., Staekenborg, S., Brunner, E., Brayne, C. and Sceltens, P. (2006) Risk of Dementia in Diabetes Mellitus : A systematic Review. *The lancet, Neurology.* 5(2), 113.

Bouzari, A., Holstege, D., and Barrett, D. M. (2015) Vitamin Retention in Eight Fruits and Vegetables: A Comparison of Refrigerated and Frozen Storage. *Journal of Agricultural and Food Chemistry.* 63(3), 957-62.

Cancer Research Uk (2018) *Alcohol Facts and Evidence.* Available from: https://www.cancerresearchuk.org/about-cancer/causes-of-cancer/alcohol-and-cancer/alcohol-facts-and-evidence#alcohol_facts5 [Accessed 31st August 2018].

Chatterjee, R., (2018) *The 4 Pillar Plan.* London, Penguin.

Daykin, N., Mansfield, L., Meads, C., julier, G., Tomlinson, A., Payne, A., Duffy, L. G., Lane, J., D'Innocenzo, G., Burnett, A., Kay, T., Dolan, P., Testoni, S., and Victor, C. (2017) What Works for Wellbeing? A Systematic Review of Wellbeing outcomes for Music and Singing in Adults. *Perspectives in Public Health.* 138(1) 39-46.

Dolson, L., (2018) How Fructose Affects your Body and health. *Verywell Fit.* Weblog Available from https://www.verywellfit.com/fructose-sweet-but-dangerous-2242217 [Accessed 27th August 2018].

Evans, C. E. L. (2017) Sugars and Health: A review of Current Evidence and Future Policy. *The Proceedings of the Nutrition Society.* 76(3), 400-407.

Ferguson, L. R. (2009) Nutrigenomics Approaches to Functional Foods. *Journal of the American Diatetic Association.* 109(3), 452-8.

German, J. B., Gibson, R. A., Krauss, R. M., nestel, P., Lamarche, B., van Steveren, W. A., Stejins, J. M., de Groot, L. C., Lock, A. L., and Destaillats, F. (2009) A Reappraisal of the Impact of Dairy Foods and Milk Fat on Cardiovascular Disease Risk. *European Journal of Nutrition.* 48(4), 191-203.

Greenbery, M. (2013) Why We Gain Weight When We're Stressed - and How Not to. *Psychology Today.* Available from https://www.psychologytoday.com/us/blog/the-mindful-self-express/201308/why-we-gain-weight-when-we-re-stressed-and-how-not [Accessed 2oth September 2018].

Grootvelt, M, Percival, B., C., and Grootveld, K. L. (2018) Chronic Non-communicable disease Risks Presented by Lipid Oxidation Products in Fried Foods. *Hepatobilliary Surgery and Nutrition*. 7(4): 305-312.

He, F. J., Li, J., and MacGregor, G. A. (2013) Effect of Longer Term Modest Salt Reduction of Blood Pressure: Cochrane Systematic Review and Meta-Analysis of Randomised Trials. *British Medical Journal (Clinical Research Ed)*. 3, 346.

Imsic, M., Winkler, S., Tomkins, B., and jones, R. (2010) Effect of Storage and Cooking on Beta-Carotene Isomers in Carrots (Daucus carota L. cv. 'Stefano'). *Journal of Agricultural and Food Chemistry*. 58(8):5109-13.

Lara-Villoslada, F., Sierra, S., Boza, J., Xaus, J and Olivares, M. (2007) Beneficial Effects of Consumption of a Dairy Product Containing two Probiotic Strains, lactobacillus coryniformis CECT5711 and Lactobacillus Gasseri CECT5714 in healthy Children. *Nutricion Hospitalaria*. 22(4), 496-502.

Jeffers, L., (2015) *Do you but pre-cut, bagged vegetables - are they just as Nutritious?* Available from https://health.clevelandclinic.org/do-you-buy-pre-cut-bagged-vegetables-are-they-just-as-nutritious/ [Accessed 20th September 2018].

Jephcote, B. (2018) Full fat milk Improves Cholesterol Levels *Diabetes.co.uk*. weblog. Available from : https://www.diabetes.co.uk/news/2018/jan/full-fat-milk-improves-cholesterol-levels-90626725.html. [Accessed 20th September 2018].

Kirk, S., Shulman, M. D., and Normal, J. (2014) Diets that Work. *The Journal of Clinical Endocrinology & Metabolism*. 99(3), 31A-32A.

Leong, K. (2013) Raw Nuts vs Roasted Nuts: Which are Better for you? *Healthy Lifestyle Docs*. Weblog. Available from : https://healthylifestyledocs.com/raw-nuts-vs-roasted-nuts-which-are-better-for-your/. [Accessed 20th September 2018].

Lewin, J. (2017) Sugar Explained. *BBC Good Food*.Weblog. Available from https://www.bbcgoodfood.com/howto/guide/sugar-explained [Accessed 20th september 2018].

Maersk, M., Belza, A., Stødkilde-Jørgensen, H., Ringgaard, S., Chavabova, E., Thomsen, H., Pederson, S. B., Astrup, A., and Richelsen, B.(2012) Sucrose-sweetened Beverages Increase Fat Storage in the Liver, Muscle, and Visceral Fat Depot: A 6-mo Randomised Intervention Study. *The American Journal of Clinical Nutrition.* 95(2), 283-289.

Matarese, L.E., Pories, J. (2014) Adult Weight Loss and Diets: Metabolic Effects and Outcomes. *Nutrition in Clinical Practice.* (6), 759-67.

Moseley, M. (2017) *Should I Worry About Arsenic in My Rice.* Available from https://www.bbc.co.uk/news/health-38910848 [Accessed 1st September 2018].

Mozaffarian, D., Katan, M. B., Ascherio, A., Stampfer, M. J. and Willett, W. C. (2006) Trans Fatty Acids and Cardiovascular Disease. *The New England Journal of Medicine.* 354(15):1601-13.

NHS (2018) *Alcohol-related Liver Disease.* Available from: https://www.nhs.uk/conditions/alcohol-related-liver-disease-arld/. [Accessed 31st August 2018].

NHS (2017) *Fat: The Facts.* Available from : https://www.nhs.uk/live-well/eat-well/different-fats-nutrition/ [Accessed 20th September 2018].

Pinnock, D. 92018) 5 ways to Improve Gut Bacteria. *The medicinal Chef.* Weblog. Available from https://www.dalepinnock.com/5-ways-improve-gut-bacteria/ [Accessed 20th September2018].

Pretorius, E. (2012) GUT Bacteria and Aspartame : Why are we Surprised? *European Journal of Clinical Nutrition.* 66, 972.

Rabin, R., C. (2016) Can you get too much Protein? *New York Times.* Available from https://www.nytimes.com/2016/12/06/well/eat/can-you-get-too-much-protein.html?_r=0 [Accessed 20th September 2018].

Rasane, P., Jha, A., Sabikhi, L., Kumar, A., and Unnikrishnan, V.S. (2015) Nutritional Advantages of Oats and Opportunities for its Processing as Value Added Foods - a Review. *Journal of food Science and Technology.* 52(2):662-675.

Silva, S., Bronze, M. R., Figueira, M. E., Siwy, J., Mischak, H., Combet, E. and Mullen, W. (2015) Impact of a 6-wk Olive Oil Supplementation in Healthy Adults on Urinary Proteomic Biomarkers of Coronary Artery Disease, Chronic Kidney Disease, and Diabetes (types 1 and 2): a Randomized, Parallel, Controlled, Double-blind Study 1–4. *American Journal of Clinical Nutrition.* 101, 44-54.

Simopoulos, A, P. (2016) An Increase in the Omega-6/Omega-3 fatty Acid ratio Increases the Risk for Obesity. *Nutrients.* 8(3): 128.

Spaeth, A. M., Dinges, D. F., and Goel, N. (2013) Effects of Experimental Sleep Restriction on Weight Gain, Caloric Intake, and meal Timing in Healthy Adults. *Sleep.* 36(7) 9810990.

Spaeth, A. M., Dinges, D. F., and Goel, N. (2015) resting Metabolic Rate Varies by Race and by Sleep deprivation. *Obesity (Silver Spring)* 23(12):2349-56.

Stevens, GA, Singh, G. M., Danaei, G, Lin, J. K., Finucane, M. M., Bahalim, A. N., Gutierrez, H. R., Cowan, M., Paciorek, C. J., Farzadfar, F., Riley, L., Ezzati, M. and Global burden of Metabolic Risk Factors of Chronic Diseases collaborating Group (Body Mass Index)(2012) National, Regional and Global Trends in Adult Overweight and Obesity Prevalences. *Population Health Metrics.* 20; 10(1):22, 10-22.

Suez, J., Korem, T., Zeevi, D., Zilberman-Schapira, G., Thaiss, C. A., Maza, O., Israeli, D., Zmora, N., Gilad, S., Weinberger, A., Kuperman, Y., Harmelin, A., Kolodkin-Gal, I., Shapiro, H., Halpern, Z., Segal, E. and

Elinav, E. (2014) Artificial Sweetener Induce Glucose Intolerance by Altering the Gut Microbiota. *Nature*. 514(7521), 181-6.

Disclaimer

I am not a trained professional, although I have done research for this book. The information in the book may not apply to everyone, particularly if you have a health condition or you are on medication. If you have any concerns speak to your GP and if you have a specific diet you have to follow then it would be wise to seek help from a nutritionist or dietitian recommended by your GP.

9 781728 649641